FIT FOR LIFE

Also available from Bantam Books

THE FIT FOR LIFE COOKBOOK
by Marilyn Diamond

Fit For Life

Harvey and Marilyn Diamond

BANTAM BOOKS

LONDON • NEW YORK • TORONTO • SYDNEY • AUCKLAND

FIT FOR LIFE
A BANTAM BOOK : 0553815881
9780553815887

Originally published in Great Britain by Bantam Books,
a division of Transworld Publishers

PRINTING HISTORY
Bantam edition published 1987
Bantam edition reissued 2004

3 5 7 9 10 8 6 4

PLEASE NOTE:
The authors do not directly or indirectly dispense medical advice or prescribe the use of diet as a form of treatment for sickness without medical approval. Nutritionists and other experts in the field of health and nutrition hold widely varying views. It is not the intent of the authors to diagnose or prescribe. The intent is only to offer health information to help you cooperate with your doctor in your mutual quest for health. In the event you use this information without your doctor's approval, you are prescribing for yourself, which is your constitutional right, but the publishers and author assume no responsibility.

Set in 11/12pt Melior by
Phoenix Typesetting, Burley-in-Wharfedale, West Yorkshire.

Bantam Books are published by Transworld Publishers,
61–63 Uxbridge Road, London W5 5SA,
a division of The Random House Group Ltd

Addresses for companies within The Random House Group Limited
can be found at:
www.randomhouse.co.uk/offices.htm

Printed and bound in Great Britain by
Cox & Wyman Ltd, Reading, Berkshire.

The Random House Group Limited makes every effort to ensure that the papers used in its books are made from trees that have been legally sourced from well-managed and credibly certified forests. Our paper procurement policy can be found at:
www.randomhouse.co.uk/paper.htm

This book is lovingly dedicated to our three wonderful children, Greg, Lisa and Beau. And to all the children of the world whose health we have an obligation to insure.

Note for readers outside the United States

You will find many fruits and vegetables mentioned in the FIT FOR LIFE eating programme. Some of these may be unfamiliar to you or unavailable in the places where you do your shopping. Remember that it is the *basic principles* of the FIT FOR LIFE plan which are important. You can achieve the same results by using fruits or vegetables which are obtainable in your area.

Pages 202–203 of FIT FOR LIFE list a wide variety of fruits, vegetables and other important stable foods. These are the vital raw materials from which the FIT FOR LIFE programme is made and co-author Marilyn Diamond has given you plenty to choose from. In some cases she mentions food stores and mail order businesses from which her American readers can obtain these products. This may not be of practical use elsewhere but remember that supermarkets and food shops everywhere are now stocking a much wider range of fruits, vegetables, and other natural products – in response to a growing demand for healthier eating.

Acknowledgments

We wish to express our deep gratitude to Joanie Prather, Robbie Levin, Russ Regan, Bonnie and M. C. Ayers, and especially to the teachers of Siddha Yoga whose combined efforts helped us make this information available to the public.

Many thanks to our editor, Patti Breitman, whose grasp, understanding, and belief in our work played such an important role in bringing this book to fruition. Also to the other editors, publicists, and staff at Warner Books whose talents, expertise, and professionalism assisted so greatly in the preparation and presentation of the book.

We also wish to thank Irene Webb and Mel Berger of the William Morris Agency for seeing the value of our work and getting others to do the same.

Special thanks also to the greatest P.R. man anywhere, anytime, Norman Winter.

Contents

Introduction *by Kay S. Lawrence, M.D.* 13
Foreword *by Edward A. Taub, M.D., F.A.A.P.* 17

PART I – The Principles

Introduction 27
1 Diets Don't Work 35
2 Natural Hygiene 40
3 The Natural Body Cycles 52
4 The Theory of Metabolic Imbalance 55
5 The Principle of High-Water-Content Food 60
6 The Principle of Proper Food Combining 74
7 The Principle of Correct Fruit Consumption 91
8 The Theory of Detoxification 110
9 Protein 119
10 Dairy Products 139
11 Exercise 151
12 You Are What You Think You Are 157
13 The Most Frequently Asked Questions 161

PART II – The Program

Introduction		183
1	Breakfast	190
2	Fresh Juices	195
3	The Energy Ladder	198
4	The FIT FOR LIFE Shopping List	200
5	The Main-Course Salad	224
6	Life-style Guidelines	229

A Four-week Example of the Fitness Life-style 235

In Conclusion 340

Bibliography 343

Index 353

Introduction

It is almost an accepted consequence of modern life that we will succumb to some type of degenerative illness sooner than we would like. However, there is also a parallel interest in finding a way to avoid what seems inevitable. As a consequence many people have quit smoking, taken up exercise, changed their diet and in general tried to take more responsibility toward prevention of illness.

The wonderful thing about the FIT FOR LIFE program is that it can be an excellent beginning along the road to health. Many people will take it up as a weight loss program, and for that it does indeed work. But more importantly it is the first step in what can be a progression to a healthier and more productive life. There are side effects to this diet: anyone who is overweight will lose weight. One will feel an increase in energy and well-being, and symptoms of disease often abate. The human body is designed for activity. Just as a muscle atrophies without use, so do all of the bodily functions. Taking drugs, eating processed foods, having a sedentary job or going everywhere by car, all cause a stagnation in certain physiological activities. The vitality and energy available as a result of eating live foods usually cause a desire for more activity. Especially if one takes up a balanced form of exercise this in turn leads to improved circulation, which is essentially the basis of health.

It is a fact that more and more people today are becoming interested in nutrition. Probably because of this there are endless books, fads and formulas on nutrition and weight loss. One can get lost and confused by all the conflicting theories. I am grateful to finally find a book that I can safely recommend to my patients.

How ironic that most things natural and normal have been labelled esoteric or put into such categories as 'alternative life-styles.' Here we have an age-old, tested and proven method of losing weight that balances natural bodily functions as well.

Society has become too technological to realize that certain primal functions are of a purely natural order and therefore wisdom is gained through their respect and study. Unfortunately in our society we respect those with degrees and status, and the more scientific and technological the data the better. The study of medicine and nutrition has also been advancing in this direction, which can sadly take us further from the truth regarding many physiological functions. For as living beings we are far more complex than the sum of our chemical reactions. It is necessary to take into account the concept of life forces and many other facets of human life which are invisible to the eye or the computer.

I find that, in some cases, the most therapeutic suggestions that I make to my patients are those that follow common sense. It doesn't sound very scientific to tell someone to take hot baths, or get more rest or recreation, or slow down their pace of life, or to eat simply so that the body is able to digest what they are eating. But these are the very suggestions that often prove to be the most effective.

The Diamonds have chosen to devote their life to the study of the human body in a way other than the two-dimensional technological approach prevalent in many universities today. That means that they have worked just as hard for their knowledge and this book proves to me their sincerity. They not only study and teach, but also live their principles.

'Modern' nutritional study has analyzed the components of the body and presumes that replacing these elements can reconstitute the same. But the common sense fact remains that it is not what's on your plate that counts, it's what you are able to use from what you eat.

The idea that we must eat a substance identical to ourselves is ludicrous. The concept of the 4 basic food groups is saying just that. 'Let's make a representation of ourselves on our plate and then eat it.'

Nutritional science is actually more complex and indeed more simple than the scientists would have us believe. It is not enough to determine levels of nutrients based on chemical data and assume that by eating something that contains these chemicals, we are being nourished. The very, very important fact is that foods must be digested in order to be used. This is why the concept of *food combining* is so very important. It allows the body to break down the foods and allow them to be assimilated into the body. Food incompletely digested is also difficult to eliminate, hence, weight gain and toxicity. I have many documented cases of patients who, by simply following proper food combining principles, have cured themselves of symptoms of disease. This has been true for almost anyone with digestive problems, but there are secondary benefits from proper digestion and elimination that have eradicated symptoms of allergies, headaches, menstrual problems, arthritis, eczema and other diseases.

The theory of food combining is a simple and practical approach to eating. By following the guide one can judge for oneself the results. I would suggest that you perform your own scientific study with your body as the laboratory. You have nothing to lose, for I have never seen anyone harmed in any way by following these guidelines of eating. Many skeptics will worry about the nutritional value of this diet because it is so different from what they have learned in grade school or seen on television commercials. But you actually have more to fear by continuing a diet that does not support your health or ideal weight. I am quite sure that you will find, as have thousands of others who follow FIT FOR LIFE, that your vitality level and sense of well-being are enhanced more and more every day, and you will feel and be healthier as a result.

Kay S. Lawrence, M.D.

Foreword

FIT FOR LIFE is a breakthrough. No guilt, no burdens, no demands. Get healthy, thin, and vibrant very soon and determine your own pace. Rush down the freeway to health, or take your time to enjoy the last of the artificial flowers along the way – the chocolates, beer, pretzels, and porterhouse steaks. It's all okay, Harvey and Marilyn Diamond tell us. Even the slightest change, the least little consistent effort, and healthy fitness ensues.

My own experience? I've lost eighteen pounds in two months. I occasionally eat fish or chicken, hardly ever succumb to beer and pretzels, and can finally see a movie without the chocolate-covered raisins in hand.

FIT FOR LIFE is an important work. It joins Ken Pelletier's *Mind as Healer, Mind as Slayer,* Harold Bloomfield and Robert Kory's *Inner Joy,* Joseph Murphy's *Power of Your Subconscious Mind,* and Norman Cousins's *Anatomy of an Illness* on the bookshelf of integrative medicine.

Integrative medicine is a new art and science based

on health promotion and 'wellness' – a natural approach to patients, regarding them not as diseases or problems, but as people needing assistance in balancing their physical, emotional, mental, and spiritual dimensions. These dimensions, when balanced or in harmony, reflect health, fitness, wholeness, and well-being – 'wellness.'

The highest calling of a physician has always been to identify the disease process at its earliest moment of inception through skill, judgment, and wisdom, and to abate the problem with surgery, medicine, or irradiation. The modern physician uses wisdom to prevent the disease process from occurring in the first place; the wellness-oriented physician works through fostering factors that contribute to homeostasis, the natural dynamic equilibrium of the body. Rather than concentrating on medicating symptoms of bodily deterioration or removing malfunctioning organs and leaving it at that, the 'wellness' physician works to assist the patient in achieving emotional calm, mental tranquillity, physical fitness, and spiritual peace.

The human body should last for 140 years, or twice as long as our present life span; so, although medical science has made great strides, it is important to remember that the job is only half done. FIT FOR LIFE and the Diamonds take us a giant step forward in extending both life's span and life's quality – a perfect example of integrative medicine. FIT FOR LIFE regards nutritional appropriateness as a matter of energy balance: Efficient absorption of food energy and efficient elimination of food bulk balance the body, and it becomes neither too thin nor too fat and retains maximum power to regain health or resist disease.

FIT FOR LIFE crushes orthodox medical dogma about the basic four food groups, milk as healthful, protein in the diet, and calorie-counting to lose weight.

Nutritional sense is a matter of monumental importance in this age of stress. 'Rechemicalization' of food with additives, preservatives, artificial flavorings, dehydration, concentration, freezing, and microwaving makes nutritional reeducation no less important than Ignaz Semmelweis's introduction of physician hand-washing before surgery or childbirth. Only 100 years have passed since that awareness descended on science. Only 100 years have passed since science stopped the bleeding, purging, and leeching that was part of our grandparents' lives. Now all our attempts at dieting and counting calories may be looked at by our grandchildren as part of our generation's folly.

FIT FOR LIFE is a perfect example of integrative medicine as an energy-based science. Both integrative medicine and this book are consumer oriented to bridge gaps between previous biological understandings and newer psychological breakthroughs that have brought out of the closet healing chemicals that our bodies produce. We are finally starting to understand how enormous are our bodies' healing powers to become well and stay healthy. Integrative medicine merges centuries of preventive medical concepts from hundreds of different cultures with the modern need to reduce stress, resolve conflict, avoid detrimental life-styles, and change behavioral patterns that lead to overweight, obesity, and then to coronary artery disease, high blood pressure, ulcers, backache, migraine, arthritis, stroke, and cancer.

Integrative medicine pursues spiritual calm, emotional peace, and physical fitness; it merges the holistic concepts of the life-styles of the Western 'lotus land' of California with the preventative medical concepts emerging from the 'Mecca' of medicine in Boston.* The Eastern doctors, traditional, with Harvard backgrounds, point out that physicians can no longer help 80 per cent of disease, that medicine and surgery still cure only 10 per cent of disease, and that the other 10 per cent of disease is now caused by accidents of surgery and side effects of medication. They proclaim the health of the American people in the 1980's to depend not on what others do for them, but on what they are willing to do for themselves. The Westerners, upstarts from UCLA, Stanford, and Berkeley, heartily agree and point consistently to laughter, hope, faith, and love as primary health ingredients. It is integrative medicine that enables the twain to meet. Integrative medicine offers patients combinations of the traditional and the holistic: diet, exercise, sunshine, rest, massage, and prayer stand alongside medication, surgical feats of derring-do, and high technology's incredible machines.

I have been honored to present integrative medicine to the California Medical Association, the American Academy of Pediatrics in Detroit, and the National Academy of Science in Washington, D.C. It is a bio-social, psycho-spiritual approach to understanding health and dealing with disease. Personal responsibility, self-value, and high regard and reverence for life are seen as primary determinants of health. Integrative medicine regards any disease as potentially reversible through the miraculous power of the body to heal itself, understands the body as an energy system, and believes

*California's best spokespeople for the holistic approach to health include Norman Cousins, George Leonard, David Harris, Charles Kleeman, M.D., Karl Pribram, M.D., Harold Bloomfield, M.D., Paul Brenner, M.D., Brugh Joy, M.D., and Ron Pion, M.D. The Boston proponents of preventative medicine include Julius Richmond, M.D., Franz Inglefinger, M.D., Rick Ingrasci, M.D., and Herbert Benson, M.D.

health is too important to leave up to science but also too important to be unscientific about.

Science is only the human mind's attempt to explain natural laws; FIT FOR LIFE explains nutrition in terms of natural laws, not what human minds have concocted up to now. When Harvey Diamond asked me to review the FIT FOR LIFE manuscript, he told me that if there was *anything,* even the slightest statement, that would offend my medical colleagues, to feel free to change it, as his purpose was to bring understanding and not resistance. Well, the book is a mind-boggler to medical theory but not an offense. It makes medical-school teaching about nutrition obsolete, even dangerous, and identifies our long-taught dogmas as merely unhealthy programming instilled by commercial interests representing milk, candy, meat, and restaurants.

To my medical colleagues I can say only that underneath the morass of chemical equations we learned was *energy.* It's all energy. The body *is* an energy system. Organs are collections of cells with identical vibrational pattems. Not only do the cells have histological similarity, they have the same energetic frequency. Homeostasis keeps it together. Disruption in cellular energy is what we label *disease.*

Energy systems function optimally with efficient fuel. Healthy, dynamic cellular equilibrium is maintained by energy intake that is equivalent to energy output. Food fuel is most efficient in the form provided by nature, since our bodies are provided by nature. There are no fields flowing with white bread. Canned, microwaved, and boiled foods are not natural. Fruit is not found naturally in sugary syrups laced with chemicals and preservatives. Streams are not filled with soft drinks. In the same way we now take food additives and junk foods for granted, for many years we took smoking for granted, and ignored its dangers. Energy provided by naturally occurring pure-state foods is the energy that is needed by naturally occurring pure-state bodies. A new wellness paradigm is now sweeping the country in a wave of consumerism attuned to jogging, aerobics, stress reduction, smoking cessation, and nutritional awareness. FIT FOR LIFE fits right in. It is an important foundation for health and future medicine – a system supporting wellness, not illness.

Edward A. Taub, M.D., F.A.A.P.
President, Foundation for Health Awareness
Assistant Clinical Professor, University of California, Irvine
Founder, Integrative Medicine

FIT FOR LIFE

PART I

The Principles

By
Harvey Diamond

Introduction

For the sake of clarity, unless otherwise noted, Harvey's voice is used in Part I and Marilyn's in Part II.

Are *you* one of those people looking for a way of living that will allow you to *sensibly* lose weight? Keep the weight off permanently? And accomplish this while experiencing all the joys of eating? If your answer to these questions is yes, then you can start to celebrate right now! Because this is the information that will enable you to do just that!

This book is the culmination of over fifteen years of intensive study of the relationship between the foods we eat and the shape of our bodies. If you are fed up with the dieting merry-go-round and are looking for some practical and sensible information that can put *you* in full control of your weight, then here is some very exciting news. You are about to learn some secrets of how to lose weight, and lose it permanently, *while eating.* I know some of you feel that's too good to be true. I felt the same way, but I found out through experience that you can indeed eat your way to the weight you wish to be.

Wouldn't it be ideal to eat and enjoy it, always feeling satisfied and not deprived, always looking forward to meals, and most important, *always* maintaining a comfortable body weight? This is what FIT FOR LIFE is all about. It is *not a diet*! It's a way of eating that can be incorporated into your life-style as a way of life, not as a dogmatic regimen. It doesn't require calorie counting; it is not a starvation diet; it avoids portion restrictions; it is not behavior modification; there are no drugs or powders; it is not a temporary measure. It is a set of dietary principles that you can use as much or as little as you wish, depending on your goals. The program puts no pressure on you. You will be comfortable all the way along, having regular, progressive success as you incorporate this information into your life.

FIT FOR LIFE brings about *permanent* results. Following its principles will teach you to stop 'living to eat' and begin 'eating to live.' It may seem as if eating great food, not counting calories, not locking up your refrigerator, and not dieting are impossible dreams, but let us assure you it is no dream – it works.

You may have reached a place in your life where you are absolutely sick and tired of hassling with your weight. You may have arrived at a position where, once and for all, *you want to find an eating program that works, that you can trust.* You want to feel confident at last that your body will be receiving all the nutrients it needs, your energy level will be high and consistent, and your weight, after a lifetime of major or even minor fluctuations, will stabilize. In short, you want to eat regularly and well, but at the same time you are determined to be free of that nagging concern over extra pounds and extra inches.

The information in this book affords you the opportunity to do all that. With this much promise, however, you may very well be thinking, 'Uh-oh, nothing but alfalfa sprouts, lettuce, and wheat germ, with a bowl of grated carrots for dessert!' *No way!* We're not from that school of thought! To put your mind at ease, let's take a look at what one typical day could include.

When you awaken in the morning, you can have a big glass of *fresh* fruit juice. Choose whatever you like, whatever is in season and most convenient for you. It can be orange, tangerine, or grapefruit juice that you make on a simple, inexpensive citrus juicer. If you happen to have one of the many all-purpose juicers on the market these days, you can make some fresh apple juice, or strawberry-apple, or watermelon, or watermelon-cantaloupe. The point is that you are encouraged to start your day with fresh juice.

If you prefer, or in addition to the juice, you can have a fresh fruit salad, or simply some fresh fruit. You can have *any* fresh fruit you like, *but no canned fruit*, and you can have as much as you feel like having. (We will explain later why canned fruit will not fit into the program.)

Perhaps you had some juice and half a cantaloupe early in the morning, and then around ten o'clock you feel hungry again. You can then have more fresh fruit, an orange or two, an apple, fresh peaches, more melon, fresh nectarines, or some cherries or grapes, depending on the season. If you have had some juicy fruit but are still feeling a little hungry, you can have a banana or two. The idea is to eat fruit during the morning, until noon, whenever you feel hungry.

At lunch you might have a big salad made with whatever fresh, raw vegetables you prefer. You can choose from a variety of dressings, and with your salad, if you wish, you might have some whole-grain toast and butter, or some soup. You might have a sandwich made from a combination of avocado, tomato, cucumber, lettuce, sprouts, and mayonnaise or butter. (By the way, if you have never had a big, luscious avocado and tomato sandwich, you are in for a real treat!)

At dinner, if you have one of those all-purpose juicers, you might want to have a big fresh vegetable-juice cocktail while you prepare the rest of your meal. You can have buttered yams, rice, or baked potatoes with an assortment of lightly steamed vegetables and salad. Or you can have a special main-course Mediterranean Rice Salad or Steak-lovers' Salad. You can have your choice of meat, chicken, or fish with vegetables and salad. For a change of pace, you might try a delicious soup with some hot buttered corn bread and coleslaw. You might have an assortment of steamed, raw, or sautéed vegetables wrapped in hot tortillas with avocado and sprouts. There are so many options and lots of new ideas to try! There is no reason to have any concern about boredom, deprivation, or confusion. You can see that there is plenty of good food to eat – exciting, delicious food, in fact! The high quality and variety of the food directly correlate with how you will look and feel. Most of the dishes you will be eating will be familiar to you, making the program easy for you to follow. And there will also be many satisfying, original meals that are new to you. Emphasizing familiar foods, the program merely calls for some very simple changes on your part.

What is completely new and different about this program is that IT IS NOT ONLY WHAT YOU EAT THAT MAKES THE DIFFERENCE, BUT ALSO OF EXTREME IMPORTANCE IS WHEN YOU EAT IT AND IN WHAT COMBINATIONS. This *when* and *how* factor is what you have been searching for, the *missing link* that will insure your success!

What is most exciting is that *this is a sensible approach to weight loss that can be readily employed as a life-style.* It works! It is innovative and it is fun!

This system will give you *lasting results*! It is **NOT** a fad diet, and it succeeds because, unlike fad diets, it is **NOT** a temporary solution! You will never again have to experience the disappointment of gaining back weight you have tried so hard to lose. You'll have at your fingertips some unique tools that you'll be able to use whenever you feel a few unwanted pounds sneaking back into your life. This system overcomes the built-in failure of fad dieting. The weight you lose on this program will be gone forever!

FIT FOR LIFE is a safe and balanced system based on natural physiological laws and cycles of the human body. And because it is based on *natural* laws, it will work for you. Everything in life is regulated by natural physical law, including your bodies, and so if we wish to lose weight effectively, we must do it in accordance with those natural laws.

At the foundation of this system is a universal truth concerning weight loss that, until now, has not been very well understood: **SAFE AND PERMANENT WEIGHT REDUCTION IS DIRECTLY RELATED TO THE AMOUNT OF VITAL ENERGY YOU HAVE AT YOUR DISPOSAL AND TO THE EFFICIENT USE OF THIS ENERGY TO ELIMINATE WASTE (EXCESS WEIGHT) FROM YOUR BODY**. The key to this system is that it works *with* your body to free up energy. With this new energy pool, your body goes to work automatically to shed any burden of excess weight. The more energy freed up, the more weight you lose. Because you will be eating to free up energy you will have more energy than you ever had before. Consistently optimizing your energy is a critical part of **FIT FOR LIFE**. It has been designed *not only* for weight loss but also for the personal energy crisis that many people are experiencing because they are continually interfering with the proper functioning of their bodies. Even if you don't need to lose weight, we assure you that on this program you will definitely be aware of a significant energy boost.

Let go of the diet mentality! If for some reason you have to get off the program, don't worry about it. Just get right back on *as soon as you can.* You can't blow this system! It is a life-style, not a temporary pattern of behavior. You can always pick it right back up at any point, and you will immediately begin to see results. Obviously, the fastest way to lose weight is not to deviate! For best results, adhere closely to the recommended program.

In the *Health Reporter* Dr. Ralph Cinque of Hygeia Health Retreat, Yorktown, Texas, writes: 'Americans have become accustomed to bulkiness, but this is by no means a universal plight. Virtually all the long-lived peoples of the world, from Asia to South America to New Zealand, tend to be lean. In America, life insurance statistics show that the greatest health, longevity and freedom from degenerative disease are found among those who are 15 per cent under the conventional standards, since the norm for body weight is too high if judged by current health standards.'

A life-style that brings on obesity is often a life-style that brings on disease. The FIT FOR LIFE program has been designed to offer a new life-style for the American people. Many of the problems of excess weight and the ill health it causes result from ignorance of how the human body works, ignorance of the critical role that energy plays in weight loss, and some very wrong ideas about how to eat. Joy Gross, in her book *Positive Power People,* tells us that 'Life is based on awesome immutable laws. Ignorance of those laws does not excuse anyone from the consequences of their non-application or the breaking of those laws.' This program is based on universal laws and physiological truths.

Apply them to your life! Reward yourself abundantly with a youthful, slender body, beauty, vitality . . . and physical, emotional, and spiritual health!

About seventeen years ago a very close friend of mine said in a moment of anger, 'Look, Blimpo, why don't you just go over there and be fat!' Blimpo? Me? This statement affected me as if someone had taken a big steel pot, put it over my head, and smashed it with a metal spoon. There were a couple of reasons that his statement so destroyed me. For one, I was certain that I was doing a fantastic job of cleverly concealing my girth with some very stylish, loose-fitting clothing, if you know what I mean. But what frustrated me more was that I had been making a career out of dieting, and my friend's comment made me realize how unsuccessful I had been. Every program that ever came down the pike, I would try. If it called for nothing but eggs and cheese for thirty days, I would do it. If it called for nothing but celery and hamburger patties for thirty days, I would eat them. And I *would* lose weight. I would lose the weight, and then as soon as the program was over, of course, I would revert to my old eating habits and go right back to my old weight. If you have ever done any dieting, you know exactly what I mean, because – let's face it – what was I thinking about while I was dieting? FOOD! As soon as the ordeal was over I would run out of the house like a scalded cat to end my deprivation. I always found that no matter how much weight I had lost, it seemed that in less time than it took me to lose it, I had already put that weight back on, plus an additional five pounds.

I hadn't been fat as a kid. But after I was released from the Air Force in my early twenties, I began to struggle with a weight problem that just wouldn't quit. During a time of my life when I should have been active and vibrant, I was nearly fifty pounds overweight. When I finally reached that much-dreaded two-hundred-pound mark and *then passed it,* I was desperate. At that same time in my life my father died at a young age, of stomach cancer. It was a terrible drawn-out ordeal, and the memory of his final days will never leave me. In his youth he had been a boxer and a longshoreman, strong and burly, over two hundred pounds. When he died he weighed under one hundred pounds. Soon after his death I awoke one night in a fever of fear, realizing that as a small-boned, 5-feet 10-inch, 202-pound male, I had all the problems that had plagued him during his life. He also was over two hundred pounds, and also like me, he had never felt really well. My subsequent studies showed me that anytime you're carrying around an extra 50 pounds, you are going to have other problems as well. My dad had frequent colds, headaches, and stomach problems. A lack of energy was his constant complaint. I had these problems too. I didn't participate in sports or social activities. Removing my shirt at the beach was always a traumatic ordeal. When I made it through my workday, I had no energy left except to eat and feel sorry for myself. (I always seemed to muster the energy necessary to eat.) When my father died I felt not only sorry for myself, but also scared.

This fear was the impetus for my turning point. My fear of dying young coupled with my desire not to be referred to as 'Blimpo' propelled me at last to a determined course of action. I was prepared to throw down my ever-present Big Mac and Coke and commit myself to the resurrection of my body. In the heat of my enthusiasm and with great resolve I plunged dramatically into a series of diets that promised to take the weight off for good. I did my first diet, then my second, then my third. After a considerable amount of frustration and disappointment I came to realize that . . .

CHAPTER 1

Diets Don't Work

One of the most ineffective and curious of all human experiences is the process of dieting. When else do people deprive and discipline themselves for days, weeks, and even months to achieve a certain goal, only to see that goal sabotaged the minute it is achieved? And as if this experience isn't frustrating enough, many dieters put themselves through this process regularly, enthusiastically losing a few pounds for a short time, only to gain them back. These dieters are draining themselves mentally, spiritually, physically, and emotionally, always searching, yet never quite finding the permanent result they seek. And this frequent, unsuccessful quest creates the undue stress and emotional havoc that dieters know too well.

What exactly is a diet, anyway? People indulge themselves and indulge themselves until they can't look at themselves in the mirror or until their clothes no longer fit. Then they grudgingly force themselves to 'diet' to make up for these past indulgences. It's like running out and locking your garage after someone has driven off in your car. It's too late; the damage is done. The 'remedy' for these indulgences is usually deprivation, and almost every one of the 'diet cures' on the market today requires the dieter to take off pounds *at any cost.* Diet schemes are an extremely expensive way to lose weight. Many times their real cost is a person's well-being.

Why don't diets work? The answer actually is quite simple. What do you think about when you're on a diet? Just as I did, you are usually thinking about what you're going to eat when the ordeal is finally over. How can you possibly succeed on your diet when all you are thinking about is food? Depriving yourself is *not* the answer to *healthy, permanent* weight loss. It usually causes you to binge later on, which complicates the problem. Deprivation and bingeing become a vicious cycle, and that's just one of the many problems with dieting.

Another is that diets are temporary; therefore, the results have to be temporary! Do you want to be permanently slim or temporarily slim? Permanent measures bring about permanent results. Temporary measures bring about temporary results. Have you ever heard anyone say, 'I've been on every diet that's ever come on the market, and nothing seems to work'? Why have they been on every diet? They've been on *every* diet without success because dieting is the wrong approach! Diets fail because of the regimentation involved. Very few of us can be regimented successfully for long when it comes to food. Yet many people, not having an alternative, continue to do what they have always done – diet – because they've never been presented with any viable alternative. They continue their search for that one panacea that will end – once and for all – their battle of the bulge.

When we go on a diet, our systems are thrown into turmoil while they try to adapt to a new regimen. They then must readapt to old patterns when the regimen ends. It's like taking a metal rod and bending it over and over again. Eventually it will become weak and break. If you jerk your body back and forth over and over again by dieting, it will become weak and break down.

But when I attack dieting, I attack an American institution. According to a Louis Harris poll, 62 per cent of all Americans are considered to be overweight. Over forty-four million Americans are considered to be clinically obese; that is, twenty pounds or more overweight. More than half of the nation is dieting or has dieted.

But the fact of the matter is that dieting doesn't work! It never has, and it never will. The sheer numbers should prove this to you. How many diets have there been over the last twenty years? Fifty? One hundred? If they really *did* work, why would there be a need for an unending chain of new ones? If diets worked, wouldn't the rate of obesity in this country be decreasing each year instead of increasing? In 1982 15 billion dollars were spent on weight-loss schemes in the United States alone. Fifteen billion dollars! If you had 15 billion dollars to spend, you could spend 1 million dollars every day for 40 years and still have 400 million dollars left over! If diets worked, that monumental amount of money would surely put an end to this problem, wouldn't it? The fact is that that incredible amount is increasing by 1 billion dollars each year. In spite of the new diets that come and go, the problem is becoming worse.

It is obvious that people have had it with the diet mentality. Confusion and frustration are rampant because most of the diets contradict one another. When the so-called authorities are at odds with one another, what is the layperson to believe? One popular diet says to eat mostly protein and very few carbohydrates. Another equally popular diet says to eat mostly carbohydrates and very little protein. Can they both be right?

Another plan says to eat whatever you feel like at the moment and then wash it out with pineapples and papayas. Yet another says to eat a small concoction of whatever you like, but be sure to exercise and be positive. One more says to eat anything you can dream of, just weigh it first. And another says you should adhere to its program for only two weeks at a time. Many diets merely rely on tedious calorie-counting. The most dangerous of all is the latest diet craze that substitutes drugs and 'nutritional powders' for real food. The cost to one's well-being from these has yet to be measured. Since we have relied on diets so heavily in the past, and we know they don't work, what now is our altemative? **YOU ARE READING IT!**

What we have here is commonsense information that people can use to determine for themselves what is best for them. It is time to take control and responsibility back from those who are arguing about who has the right answer. What we have is a new approach, a new way of thinking, *a new way of eating*, so that diets become unnecessary and as obsolete as sealing wax. It is obvious that diets are not working, so let's get rid of them and set ourselves free! Why not find out firsthand that the only *permanent* results you will see in weight loss will come when you **STOP DIETING!**

That's what I did. I finally had had it. I finally gave up dieting. I resolved to find an answer that would make sense to me, that would be reasonable and permanent. After three years of driving myself crazy with diets, it became obvious that what I needed was to learn how to properly take care of my body. What I wanted to find was a course of study that would teach me how to acquire and maintain that slim and healthy body that I *knew* was inside of me.

One evening at a music festival 2,000 miles from home, I overheard two rather healthy-looking individuals discussing the idiosyncracies of a friend in Santa Barbara, California, referring to his long dissertations on the beauty of good health. My ears perked up. 'Excuse me,' I interrupted, 'who is this fellow you are discussing?' In less than twenty-four hours I was on my way to Santa Barbara. Little did I know that I was on the brink of one of the most remarkable discoveries of my life. I was about to be introduced to a most extraordinary, age-old science known as . . .

CHAPTER 2

Natural Hygiene

Natural Hygiene – when I first heard the term, I thought, Yeah, I know what that is, brushing my teeth and being sure to wash behind my ears. As it happens, that is what many people think when they hear this term. Actually Natural Hygiene is a most remarkable approach to the care and upkeep of the human body. The first time I heard the term, I was staring into the face of the healthiest person *I* had ever met. One look at him and I knew he *had* to know something about how to take care of his body. As I looked at his clear eyes, radiant skin, serene demeanor, and well-proportioned body, I could not help but reflect on all of the health professionals I had sought advice from in the past who did not exemplify the physical ideal any more than I did. When he met me, he said, 'You know, you're killing yourself and you don't have to be.' Well, I lit right up like a Christmas tree. That sentence was my introduction to Natural Hygiene and the beginning of a most rewarding friendship. In a matter of hours Mr. Jensen (pseudonym used per request) explained to me in a most concise, easy-to-understand way exactly why I was fat and why I was having such a struggle losing weight and keeping it off. It all made so much sense to me that I was dumbfounded at its obvious simplicity. Listening to this initial explanation of how to achieve and maintain a truly fit body I could be proud of, I was filled with a sense of joy and relief I had never before known. Here was the information that I had known I would somehow find.

I had the very good fortune to study with Mr. Jensen for the next three and a half years. And what an eye-opening experience it was! Not only did I have the daily benefit of his knowledge, but I acquired and read everything I could find on the subject of Natural Hygiene. I determined that the study, practice, and teaching of Natural Hygiene were going to be my life's work. After leaving Santa Barbara, I studied Natural Hygiene intensely for the next 10 years. For several years I counseled people privately on how to use the principles of Natural Hygiene as a life-style, and I continue to do so. In 1981 I began a seminar program known as THE DIAMOND METHOD, and between then and now I have spoken to many thousands of people. The hundreds of enthusiastic letters I received from people of all walks of life and all ages attest to the effectiveness of this way of eating. Early in 1983 I received a doctorate in nutritional science from the American College of Health Science in Austin, Texas, the only institution in the United States to grant a degree in Natural Hygiene.

One month after being introduced to Natural Hygiene, I had lost the 50 pounds that I had been wrestling with for so long. That was in 1970. I have not put any of that weight back on in all this time. And I love to eat. I'm one of those people who can put on a few pounds just by reading *Gourmet* magazine. The difference now, however, is that I have learned *how* to eat so I not only satisfy my *desire* to eat but also assist my body in maintaining itself at the weight that is most becoming to me. I've learned to eat to live, not live to eat. In other words, I have not put the weight back on in all this time because I did not take it off with a diet! I altered my eating habits. That's what did it.

Mind you, the loss of weight is only one of the benefits of the incorporation of Natural Hygiene as a life-style. A phenomenal increase in my energy and an overall feeling of well-being have also become welcome additions to my life. I never dreamed I could experience such a consistently high level of energy. I have such a surplus of energy all the time now, that some of my acquaintances find me annoying! As I pass 40 years of age, I cannot help but be delighted at how much healthier I am now than I was when 25! And I owe it to Natural Hygiene.

Natural Hygiene can trace its history to early Greece. Four hundred years before the birth of Christ, Hippocrates stated its philosophy accurately when he taught: 'Thy food shall be thy remedy.' The modern history of Natural Hygiene in the United States began in 1830, when an organization was formed called the American Physiological Society. Eight years later it established a library and provisions store in Boston, which could properly be called the country's first health food store.

Around 1850 four medical doctors, Sylvester Graham, William Alcott, Mary Gove, and Isaac Jennings, began the first major modern Natural Hygiene movement. Quickly many other members of the medical profession joined their ranks, wishing to add a more natural approach to traditional medicine. In 1862 Dr Russell Trall formed a national hygienic association. In 1872 Dr Trall published *The Hygienic System*, a work that was very well received. It preceded many works on Natural Hygiene, all of which taught the importance of diet in acquiring and maintaining a high level of health.

One of the most well-respected and knowledgeable Natural Hygienists of our time is Dr Herbert M. Shelton, now retired, who from 1928 to 1981 ran a 'health school' including a clinic, laboratory, and teaching program in San Antonio, Texas. Dr Shelton is generally considered to be the greatest oracle of Natural Hygienic philosophy, principles, and practice. He produced a wealth of literature with new findings and thoughts, and he added more to the science and art of Natural Hygiene than any other person. In Dr Shelton's words: 'The laws of nature, the truths of the universe, the principles of science, are just as certain, as fixed and immutable, in relation to health as they are in relation to all things else. Natural Hygiene is that branch of biology which investigates and applies the conditions upon which life and health depend, and the means by which health is sustained in all its virtue and purity, and restored when it has been lost or impaired.'

Today's most eminent, active proponent of Natural Hygiene is most certainly T. C. Fry, the dean of the American College of Health Science, a most brilliant spokesperson for health. In his words, 'Natural Hygiene is in harmony with nature, in accord with the principles of vital, organic existence, correct in science, sound in philosophy and ethics, in agreement with common sense, successful in practice, and a blessing to humankind.' His credo is 'Health is produced only by healthful living.'

Dr K. R. Sidhwa, a leading Natural Hygienist in London, recently described Natural Hygiene at the Third World Congress of Alternative Medicine as 'the ultimate healing philosophy or technique.'

Natural Hygiene is practiced today by people around the world who enjoy long, healthy, disease-free lives. For information about Natural Hygiene or to receive the society's periodical, write to The American Natural

Hygiene Society, Drawer A, Box 30630, Tampa, Florida 33630. In Canada the address is The Canadian Natural Hygiene Society, P.O. Box 235, Station T, Toronto, Ontario, Canada M6B 4A1.

What precisely does 'Natural Hygiene' mean? You were on the right track in the beginning if you thought of cleaning your teeth. The word *hygiene* connotes cleanliness. The word *natural* implies a process unhampered by artificial forces. **THE BASIC FOUNDATION OF NATURAL HYGIENE IS THAT THE BODY IS ALWAYS STRIVING FOR HEALTH AND THAT IT ACHIEVES THIS BY CONTINUOUSLY CLEANSING ITSELF OF DELETERIOUS WASTE MATERIAL.** It is the approach of understanding the effect that food has on the length and quality of one's life. Its focus is on prevention and healthful living. It teaches people how to eliminate the *cause* of their health problems rather than constantly battle the effects of continual violation of natural laws.

The underlying basis of Natural Hygiene is that the body is self-cleansing, self-healing, and self-maintaining. Natural Hygiene is based on the idea that all the healing power of the universe is within the human body; that nature is always correct and cannot be improved upon. Therefore, nature does not seek to thwart any of its own operations. We experience problems of ill health (i.e., excess weight, pain, stress) only when we break the natural laws of life.

The most beautiful thing about Natural Hygiene is that it affords you the opportunity to control your weight by supplying you with useful tools. Some of these tools are inborn: common sense, instincts, logic, and reasoning. These are critical tools that we all have built-in, but for one reason or another as life goes on we rely less and less on these attributes. I can't count how many times I have heard people say, after hearing how Natural Hygiene explains a certain situation, 'You know, I always kind of felt that's how it should be, but . . .' Their instincts were telling them one thing, but outside pressures convinced them to do otherwise. Through the passage of time their instincts were heeded less and less until they were not given notice at all. Many examples of how to use common sense, instincts, and logic to control your body weight will be presented throughout this book.

The greatest tool of all – indeed, the greatest gift of all – is the human body and the immense intelligence that directs it. The human body has to be nature's finest creation. It is unmatched in power, capacity, and adaptability. The intelligence inherent in our bodies is so vast that it is positively staggering. The human heart beats about one hundred thousand times every 24 hours. Consider the fact that the heart and its pumping system, which scientists have attempted to duplicate without success, pump 6 quarts of blood through over *ninety-six thousand miles* of blood vessels. This is an equivalent of 6,300 gallons being pumped *per day*. That is almost one hundred fifteen million gallons in only 50 years.

The 6 quarts of blood are made up of over twenty-four trillion cells that make three to five thousand trips throughout the body *every day*. Seven million new blood cells are produced every second! This pumping system has the capability of working *nonstop* for decades without skipping a beat. And this is only the circulatory system!

Consider the heat this machine must generate in accomplishing these functions, yet realize that it maintains a constant temperature of around 98.6 degrees! The biggest organ of the body, the skin, is made up of over four million pores that are constantly acting as the cooling system for this machine. The digestive and metabolic systems have the remarkable ability to transform the food we eat into healthy blood, bone, and cell structure. Perfect balance is always maintained, and if it were off by only a small fraction, the balance would be destroyed. The lungs succeed in supplying the blood with the oxygen it needs. A complex skeletal system furnishes a supporting framework to allow the body to stand upright and walk. The skeletal system works in harmony with an amazing muscular system that allows locomotion.

This machine can astonishingly reproduce itself! The force and wisdom necessary to turn a fertilized ovum into a fully grown man or woman are beyond our comprehension. The five senses alone can stun the intellect. The list of activities performed by your body on a regular basis could fill a book. At the helm of this pinnacle of perfection is the brain, overseeing all these miraculous activities, making sure everything is working with a precision that would make the work of a master watchmaker look clumsy. The brain consists of more than twenty-five billion cells that are the most highly developed of any known.

Looking at an individual cell, you will be even more impressed. A single cell cannot be seen without a microscope, yet what goes on within a cell is astounding. The wisdom of a single cell is said to exceed all the accumulated knowledge of the human race to date. Even the smallest cell in your body is about one billion times the size of its smallest component! The cell is the site of more chemical reactions than all the chemical factories in the world combined. There are thousands of components in a cell: chromosomes, genes, DNA, organelles, mitochondria, enzymes, hormones, amino acids, and thousands of various chemicals and compounds too numerous to mention. And no one on this earth can explain what makes an individual cell operate. All the thousands of different functions can be categorized, but the force behind these functions is beyond our comprehension. In other words, the innate intelligence of the body is infinitely more sophisticated than our thinking minds. And to think there are over seventy-five trillion (75,000,000,000,000) of these astounding cells working with pinpoint perfection for some sixty, seventy, eighty years, or more!

Inside each cell is a nucleus that contains chromosomes that contain genes. And inside genes is the stuff of life: DNA. DNA is what determines what color your eyes are, or what fragrance a flower will have, or the iridescence of a bird's feathers. If you took all the DNA from all the genes of all your 75 trillion cells, it would fit into a box the size of an ice cube. Yet if all this DNA were unwound and joined together, the string would stretch from the earth to the sun and back more than four hundred times! That's almost eighty billion miles!

Let's use an analogy to help you understand the size of the numbers we are talking about and what cooperation of titanic proportions is necessary to coordinate them. Consider that there are some four billion inhabitants of the earth. Now, I realize that it would be difficult to envision even a few million of those inhabitants getting together and cooperating harmoniously *in all things.* If that seems difficult, then imagine all four billion individuals on earth acting in unison. As impossible as it seems, compared with the inner workings of the body, that is nothing! Imagine 18,000 earths, *each* with 4 billion inhabitants and every last one acting in unison. All have the same political beliefs, the same religious beliefs, and the same intellectual beliefs, and all are working for the exact same goals. Ha! There's more of a chance of the moon being made of green cheese. But that is precisely what the trillions of cells in your body do every day!

One human cell in the laboratory, free from all bodily influences, will divide some fifty times before dying. If all our cells divided that often, we would reach a weight of more than eighty trillion tons! Only with such staggering thoughts as these is it possible to grasp some idea of the infinite intelligence necessary to coordinate the activities of such an astronomical number of cooperating cells.

As one last illustration, imagine yourself writing an extremely important letter to a friend, while simultaneously watching your favorite TV program *and* listening to a positive-mental-attitude tape. How well will you perform these three functions? Probably not too well. Now, at the same time, prepare your dinner and wash the floor. Forget it. Trying to do these five tasks at the same time leaves no chance for any of them to be performed with any high level of efficiency. And that's only five activities. Your body is performing quadrillions of processes twenty-four hours a day! Not millions or billions or even trillions, but *quadrillions*! And not haphazardly, but with pinpoint perfection, carrying on all the metabolic and life-sustaining processes of your existence. When we view the vastness of the human body's faculties and processes, we must stand in awe of the enormous intelligence displayed.

Considering these facts, is it at all conceivable that this truly magnificent machine would be left without the mechanism to achieve a proper body weight? *No!* It is inconceivable. Mechanisms for the body's self-preservation are built in at birth. **HEALTH IS YOUR BIRTHRIGHT, AND BEING OVERWEIGHT IS NOT HEALTH.** The same way a plant will reach for the light source from wherever it is located in a room, so your body will forever strive for perfection. As an automatic biological process of existence, just like breathing and blinking your eyes, the human body ceaselessly strives to be fit. *The secret is to learn how to facilitate the process rather than thwart it.* Every way we interact with our environment affects our well-being, but in no other area of life are our biological needs violated more flagrantly than in our diets. If you have a weight problem, there is no question that the food you are putting into your body is the major factor contributing to that problem. From every area of the healing profession, more and more information is coming to light concerning the relationship of food to your well-being.

A letter from Dr David Reuben to his fellow physicians in his best-selling book *Everything You Always Wanted to Know About Nutrition* said, 'There is a whole category of substances that have a far more intense effect on our patients than drugs. That category is food – and through no fault of our own, we have neglected that particular area of medicine. Our medical education neglected it, our internships neglected it, and our residencies neglected it. And for good reason – we had to take care of great masses of sick people.

'But now it is becoming obvious, with each successive issue of our most responsible medical journals, that many of these "sick people" are sick specifically because of what they are eating – or not eating.' He then added, 'People of America, the greatest threat to the survival of you and your children is not some terrible nuclear weapon. *It is what you are going to eat from your dinner plate tonight.*'

The *Dietary Goals for the United States,* prepared by the staff of the Select Committee on Nutrition and Human Needs, United States Senate, states: 'As a nation we have come to believe that medicine and medical technology can solve our major health problems. The role of such important factors as diet in cancer and heart disease has long been obscured by the emphasis on the conquest of these diseases through the miracles of modern medicine. Treatment, not prevention, has been the order of the day.

'The problems can never be solved merely by more and more medical care. The health of individuals and the health of the population is determined by a variety of biological, behavioral, and environmental factors. *None of these is more important than the foods we eat!*'

If it can be assumed that the incidence of the number-one and number-two killer diseases (heart disease and cancer) in this country can be decreased by people knowing how and what to eat, imagine what it could do for the problem of overweight, often a precursor to these killers. How fortunate! Now that it is finally apparent that the foods we eat, obesity, and degenerative diseases are very much interrelated, we can relate that discovery to an entire field of knowledge devoted to the effect of food on the human body.

It is interesting that the field of Natural Hygiene has existed in this country and been utilized by thousands of people for over a century and a half, and yet very few people have even heard of it. Very possibly *you* have never heard of it prior to this introduction. During my seminars I ask every audience, 'How many of you have ever heard of Natural Hygiene?' *Less than one per cent ever raise their hands!* It is strange that such a simple, practical, and *successful* area of health care is so unknown. Aside from its not receiving very much attention in the media, the reason for its obscurity is that its principles have never before been capsulized into a viable program for people to utilize.

What Marilyn and I have done is synthesize the basic fundamentals of Natural Hygiene into a series of commonsense, easy-to-follow dietary principles that facilitate the goal of eliminating obesity and alleviate the necessity for dieting. According to Jack D. Trop, past president of the American Natural Hygiene Society (which was formed in 1948): FIT FOR LIFE 'simplifies the basic fundamentals of Natural Hygiene and brings them to a large public forum for the first time in history.'

Natural Hygiene is a vast subject with a tremendous amount to offer the serious student. For some in-depth material, books, periodicals, and, in my opinion, the finest correspondence course on Natural Hygiene available anywhere, contact the American College of Health Science, 6600-D Burleson Road, Austin, Texas 78744.

Going a little deeper now into the philosophy of Natural Hygiene, let's take a look at one of the more interesting phenomena of the human body. An introduction to this phenomenon is necessary to learn how to take weight off easily and permanently. In all likelihood, though you may have dieted extensively in the past, you have probably never come into contact with a fascinating and intriguing concept known as . . .

CHAPTER 3

The Natural Body Cycles

A BRIEF INTRODUCTION

What are these cycles? Most people are not even aware that they exist! Yet extensive research on these physiological cycles has been done, most notably by the Swedish scientist Are Waerland, by T. C. Fry of the American College of Health Science, in writings on biological clocks by psychologist Gay Gaer-Luce, and by myriad researchers and scientists in their studies of the circadian rhythms. Information from these sources is the basis for our suggestion that the human's ability to deal with food relies on the effective functioning of three regular daily cycles.

These cycles are based on rather obvious functions of the body. To put it in its simplest terms, on a daily basis we take in food (appropriation), we absorb and use some of that food (assimilation), and we get rid of what we don't use (elimination). Although each of these three functions is always going on to some extent, each is more intense during certain hours of the day.

noon to 8 p.m. – **APPROPRIATION** (eating and digestion)

8 p.m. to 4 a.m.	– **ASSIMILATION**	(absorption and use)
4 a.m. to noon	– **ELIMINATION**	(of body wastes and food debris)

Our body cycles can become apparent to us if we simply witness our bodies in action. Obviously, during our waking hours we eat (appropriate), and if we put off eating, our hunger tends to heighten as the day goes on. When we are sleeping and the body has no other noticeable work to do, it is assimilating what was taken in during the day. When we awaken in the morning, we have what is called 'morning breath' and perhaps a coated tongue because our bodies are in the midst of eliminating that which was not used – body wastes.

Did you ever notice what happens if you eat late at night? How do you feel the next morning? When you awaken, you feel groggy or 'drugged.' The assimilation cycle that proceeds *after* food has left the stomach has been thwarted. Physiologically our bodies want to eat early in the evening so that at least three hours can pass, the time needed for food to leave the stomach, and the assimilation cycle can start on time. Since the food is not yet digested, because you have eaten late at night, it is not ready to be assimilated. You have extended the appropriation cycle far beyond its limit, and you have postponed the assimilation cycle well into the time when the body wants to be eliminating. The regular eight-hour cycles have now been thrown into turmoil. The natural workings of your body have been thwarted; thus you awaken feeling 'drugged.' Similarly, if you have ever skipped breakfast, you have probably made it until lunch because your body was eliminating and didn't want to eat anyway. Going later than lunch without food, however, would be uncomfortable because your body had entered the appropriation cycle and was prepared to take in food.

This program has been designed to *return* you to a life-style that is based on your natural body cycles. As we proceed and you become more familiar with the principles that are the basis of the program, the usefulness of the body cycles will become increasingly apparent. But for now it is sufficient to understand that those of us who are waging the battle of the bulge should be most concerned with the elimination cycle. If that cycle is facilitated, rather than thwarted, your success in releasing the thin body locked within you can practically be guaranteed. Understand that elimination means the removal of toxic waste and excess weight from your body. The reason that 62 per cent of the people in this country are overweight is that our traditional eating habits have consistently obstructed the all-important elimination cycle. In other words, we have been taking food in (at a record pace!), we have been using what we need from that food, but we have NOT been getting rid of what we can't use. Since so many Americans eat a hearty breakfast, a hearty lunch, and a hearty dinner, far more time is spent appropriating than eliminating. Is it any wonder that so many of us are carrying around so much excess weight?

So to lose weight, the secret of success is getting rid of the toxic wastes and excesses we carry around. Where does this toxic waste come from in the first place, and how does one get rid of it? According to Natural Hygiene, the explanation for why a person has a weight problem is . . .

CHAPTER 4

The Theory of Metabolic Imbalance

Toxemia – the term used by Natural Hygiene pioneers to describe what modern science now calls metabolic imbalance – was first written about by John H. Tilden, M.D. The human body is finely designed to stay in balance in terms of tissue building up (anabolism) and tissue breaking down (catabolism). An excess of one over the other is metabolic imbalance.

In 1926 Dr Tilden wrote a book entitled *Toxemia Explained.* Unlike all the 'diet' books I had read, this was the first source that gave me a clear understanding of how my body worked and exactly *why* it did not seem to want to cooperate with me in terms of my weight. In the most easy-to-understand way it explained what was wrong, why it was wrong, what to do about it, and how to do it! For the first time I had the feeling that I could be successful in turning my waddle into a walk. Although this book addressed itself to the entire subject of health, it supplied what I needed to know quite specifically about **WHY ONE GETS FAT!**

There have been many books subsequently written on toxemia, but Dr Tilden's book is considered the tour de force in the field of Natural Hygiene. Dr. Tilden explains that a situation of toxemia in the system lays the foundation for putting on excess weight. By keeping your system toxin-free you significantly increase your chance of having a comfortable body weight, because excesses of toxins in the body are the forerunners of obesity.

So, what is toxemia? Where does it come from? And what can one do to minimize it? According to the precepts of Natural Hygiene, there are two basic ways it is produced in the system. One is a normal, natural function of the body; the other we regularly contribute to, either knowingly or not. Both demand energy for its removal from your body.

The first way toxemia is produced is through the process of metabolism. As you are reading this page your inner body is not still; it is hard at work. Old cells are constantly being replaced by new cells. In fact, three hundred billion to eight hundred billion old cells a day are replaced with new ones.[1] These old cells are toxic (poisonous) and must be removed from your system as soon as possible by one of the four channels of elimination: bowels, bladder, lungs, or skin. This is a normal, natural process of the body and is not something with which to concern yourself *unless* for some reason this toxic waste material is *not* eliminated at the same rate that it is being produced. *As long as there is a sufficient amount of energy at the body's disposal*, this waste *is* eliminated properly.

The second way toxemia is produced in the system is from the by-products of foods that are not properly digested, *assimilated*, and incorporated into cell struc-

[1] The number of cells that need to be replaced each day depends on how much cooked or caustic food is in the diet, causing cells to be lost from the alimentary canal.

ture. In this country we have the most peculiar habit of altering practically everything we eat from its original state before eating it. Rather than a sufficient quantity of fresh foods dominating our dietary intake, the major portion of what we eat is processed. If it isn't processed to death before we get our hands on it, we alter it in some way ourselves. We fry, barbecue, steam, sauté, stew, boil, or broil almost all the food we eat. Because the food has been altered from its original state and we are not biologically adapted to deal with so much of this altered food, the by-products of its incomplete digestion and assimilation form a certain amount of residue in the body. This residue is toxic. If these types of foods PREDOMINATE in one's diet, *the system is overtaxed on a regular basis.*

So your body is building toxemia daily in two ways: through the normal process of metabolism and by the residue left over from the foods not efficiently utilized. As far as your weight is concerned, common sense will tell you that if more of this toxic waste is built than is eliminated, there is going to be a buildup of the excess. That translates as *overweight.* Adding to the problem, toxins are of an acid nature. When there is an acid buildup in the body, the system retains water to neutralize it, adding even more weight and bloat.

Imagine working in a large corporation where your job is to shred twenty boxes of written material and throw it away every day. Now let's say that because either you don't have enough time or you don't have enough energy, or both, you can shred only fifteen boxes a day. That means the next day you'll be delivered another twenty boxes – but you still have five boxes left over from the previous day. Being able to shred only fifteen, you will have ten extra boxes after the second day. If you started on Monday and worked seven days a week, on the second Monday of your job after your delivery of twenty boxes, you will have a total of fifty-five boxes and be capable of dealing with only fifteen! After only one week you have forty extra boxes. These will have to be stored somewhere until they can be shredded. But where? If you have any kind of weight problem, the above predicament is exactly what your body has to deal with. If you build more toxic waste every day than is eliminated from your body, then it is going to be stored somewhere. Your body, ever attempting to protect itself and maintain its integrity, tends not to store this waste in or near the vital organs. It will be stored in the fatty tissue and the muscles. That means in the thighs, in the buttocks, around the midsection, in the upper arms, under the chin – all those places where we lament the bulges most. If the problem goes unchecked, the ultimate result is not only obesity but general discomfort and lethargy as the body expends a great deal of its energy in an attempt to rid itself of this accumulated toxic waste.

What Dr Tilden was relating to his readers over half a century ago was this: Although the problem appears to be out of the individual's control, it is not! It is a simple physiological phenomenon that is not a mystery. Anyone can take control of the situation and direct it to whatever degree he or she desires. It is simply a matter of understanding toxemia and doing what is necessary to remove the toxic waste that already exists in one's body and see that it is not accumulated at a more rapid pace than it is eliminated.

Having this understanding, can you now see the extreme importance of your elimination cycle being allowed to operate uninterrupted with the utmost efficiency? Can you see how if you interfere even unknowingly with your elimination cycle, you are going to force your body to retain and store the toxic waste that is the beginning of a weight problem?

Of course, stating that all one has to do is remove toxins from the body and not build them back up is all well and good, but exactly how is this accomplished? This was our concern. This is what we saw could be developed out of my study of Natural Hygiene: A convenient life-style based on the understanding of how to continuously cleanse the body of its toxic waste and never allow it to build to an unacceptable level. The most beautiful thing is that it's fun, not restrictive. Eating remains a joy; it does not become a clinical endeavor. This is a must for me personally, since I could never embrace an approach to eating that deprived my gourmet palate.

That was what prompted my wife, Marilyn, to put her gourmet background to work and develop an approach to food preparation that would enhance the program and turn it into a truly delightful eating life-style (which will be presented to you in Part II).

So how do we maintain metabolic balance and accomplish the removal of toxic waste from the system while still enjoying our food? There are three easy-to-understand and easy-to-follow principles, or tools, that can assist you in doing precisely that. The first of these critical and vital tools that can help you realize your goal of *permanent* weight loss is . . .

CHAPTER 5

The Principle of High-Water-Content Food

Before describing this principle, I would like to invite you to participate in a simple and interesting exercise. List on a piece of paper *everything* you ate today. If you haven't yet eaten your day's fare, list everything you ate yesterday. By the end of this chapter the list will serve as a powerful tool in making a certain important point. In listing the foods eaten, list everything, even 'tastes' of things; e.g., your friend made her famous soufflé and you had just one little bite. If you can remember, list everything to enter your body. Now put the list away for a while, and let's get on with this principle.

As an absolute prerequisite of life, water is right up there with food and air. From the moment you are born until you leave this planet, your body instinctively craves food, air, and water for your survival. You know what happens to a plant when it is deprived of water. It wilts and dies. The same would happen to your body if it were deprived of water. Its importance is clear.

What do I mean when I say high-water-content food? Consider that we're living on a planet that is over 70 per cent water. If you were on the moon looking down on earth, you would see that 71 per cent of the surface of our planet is water. The other 29 per cent is land. Everything is a microcosm of a macrocosm. If you go deeper into the planet and look at the animals of the class Mammalia, you will find out that our bodies are 70 per cent water, at least! When I first heard that, I found it very hard to believe. I couldn't see any, nor could I even hear it in movement. But 70 per cent of the human body is indeed made up of water. Now let me ask you a common-sense question. (And this is what Natural Hygiene is about. It's making use of your inborn sense of what is right.) If the planet earth is 70 per cent water, and depends upon that amount of water for its survival, and your body is 70 per cent water does it not make sense that for you to maintain a body that is always in its best condition, you must consume a diet that is at least 70 per cent water? If your body is 70 per cent water, then where will it get that water if you don't replenish it on a regular basis? From the moment you are born until the last breath you take your body is craving this essential of life. You must have water for survival. *I am not talking about drinking water.*

Some people might be saying right now, 'Hey, that's great, I drink my eight glasses of water a day.' But in no way will drinking water bring you the success I am referring to. When I say high-water-content food, I am talking about two foods grown on this planet that naturally have a very high water content. Only two foods meet that requirement. They are fruits and vegetables. Anything else you eat is a concentrated food. *Concentrated* means that the water content has been removed, either by processing or cooking. I am *not* saying you have to eat exclusively fruits and vegetables to lose the weight you want to lose. What I *am* saying is that since our bodies are 70 per cent water, we should be eating a diet that is approximately 70 per cent water content, and that means fruits and vegetables should PREDOMINATE in our diets. The other 30 per cent will consist of the concentrated foods: breads, grains, meat, dairy products, legumes, and so on.

There are two extremely important reasons why we need this water, and they're the same two reasons why drinking water will not fill the bill: *nourishment and cleansing of the organism.* Water transports the nutrients in food to all the body's cells and in turn removes toxic wastes.

All the nutritional requirements that the human body has – all the vitamins, minerals, proteins, amino acids, enzymes, carbohydrates, and fatty acids that exist, that the human body needs to survive – are to be found in fruits and vegetables. The nutritional requirements are carried by the water in those fruits and vegetables into your intestines, where all nutrition is absorbed. If you are eating foods high in water content, that means you are eating foods that have all of the requirements of the human body. Some of you might be saying, 'Well, I take vitamin-mineral supplements.' That's not what we're talking about. The vitamins and minerals that I am talking about, that are usable by the human body, are to be found in abundance in orchards and gardens, not in drugstores.

Besides carrying nutrients into the body, this water performs the essential function of cleansing the body of wastes. For our purposes, cleansing and detoxifying are the same. In the quest to lose weight, this cleansing or detoxification is of paramount importance. Everything you have, no matter what it is, has to be washed if you want it to be clean. In all likelihood, you took a bath or shower today. If you didn't, well, then you probably took one yesterday or will take one tomorrow. It's only going to be so long before you take a bath or shower, because you want to be clean. Same with your clothes. What if the clothes that you're wearing right now were not removed from your body for six months! You know, of course, that I'm being facetious when I say that. You wouldn't do that, because the clothes would become so foul that you would not be able to go near anyone. What if you didn't wash your car for six months and it didn't rain? You would not be able to see through the window to drive. That is how dirty it would become. That is how dirty anything would become if it is not washed.

Guess what one thing is not being washed and cleansed on a regular basis in this country? The insides of our bodies! We eat and live in such a way as to never allow the insides of our bodies to be cleansed sufficiently, and that is why 62 per cent of the population of this country is overweight. It is also a contributing factor to the fact that three out of four people in this country will develop some form of heart disease or cancer in their lifetime. The outside of the body is washed, but the inside, which is far more important, is *not* washed. I'm talking about some people going for *decades,* **THEIR ENTIRE LIVES**, without ever doing what is necessary to wash out the toxic waste from inside their bodies. The only way this can be done is by eating foods that are high in water content. Drinking water won't do it, because drinking water does not carry the enzymes and other life-preserving elements into the body that the water in fruits and vegetables does. **ALL THREE OF OUR BODY CYCLES FUNCTION WITH THE GREATEST EASE WHEN SUPPLIED WITH THIS WATER ON A REGULAR BASIS.**

It's interesting that we eat in such a way as to *not* cleanse but pollute our bodies. We eat in such a way as to *clog* them. We don't want to be clogged up any further, because the more we clog ourselves, the more we're going to put on weight, and the more difficult it will be to get that weight off. In fact, from now on when you look at the foods that you are about to eat, do just that – *look* at the plate of food that you're going to put into your body, and simply ask yourself this question: 'Is this food that I'm going to put into this magnificent, intelligent body of mine going to cleanse me, or is it going to clog me?' Stated another way: 'Is this meal predominated by fruits and vegetables?' This is a very important question to ask yourself regularly. It's very simple. Am I eating a food right now that's going to cleanse me (detoxify me), or is it going to clog me?

Most of the food we eat in this country is of a clogging nature. Our food clogs our bodies, and then, because we're clogged, we start to feel bad and we take measures to feel better, but at the same time we're still eating foods that are clogging up the system. So, from now on ask yourself, when you look at a meal, 'Is approximately 70 per cent of this meal of a high-water-content nature?' Because I will tell you something without reservation: If it's not, there is no way in the world you are going to successfully lose the weight you want to lose and keep it off permanently. If you truly want to be healthy and experience the body that you know you deserve to have, then it is an absolute prerequisite that you ask yourself this question. The reason there are 200,000 heart bypass operations in this country every year is because people's arteries are *clogged*! I would be willing to wager that few, if any, of these unfortunate 200,000 were on a diet predominated by high-water-content food. It's odd, but the things we receive for free we abuse the most. Because we are given these miraculous, incredible bodies at birth for free, we tend to take them for granted and abuse them. We must work *with* our bodies, not against them. One perfect way to do that is to cleanse them, not clog them.

The reason we eat so much food that is clogging

rather than cleansing is that we're prisoners. Prisoners! That's right. We're prisoners of our taste buds. We will do anything for our taste buds. If there is a food that can't outrun us, and it's not nailed down, and it will fit into our mouths, and it tastes good, we'll eat it! We don't think twice about it. The only requirement we have about food is 'How does it taste?' But what about the rest of the body? When you look at the tiny area of the body that your taste buds occupy, and then you look at the rest of your body (which is what has to deal with the foods that pass over your taste buds) you have to wonder why people place so much attention on one small part of the body and ignore such a large part.

How many times have you heard someone say, 'You know what, I woke up this morning, I was real late, I didn't have a chance to take a bite before I went out of the house. I ran out of the house to the office. I had more work than I could possibly take care of, I never took a coffee break. I never took a lunch break. I worked straight all day long.' You've probably heard that part before. But now five o'clock rolls around; it's time to go home. All of a sudden this person realizes how hungry he really is. He's rubbing his stomach and saying, 'Man, am I hungry. I haven't eaten all day. I'm going out right now to get myself something that's going to wash out my intestines and cleanse my colon.' No way! That is not what you've heard. It's more like 'I'm going to get myself a pizza or a cheeseburger.' The thing that people do when they're hungry, most of the time, is decide what is going to taste best and then go and eat that food. If you think exclusively of what is going to taste good, your body never has the opportunity to cleanse or detoxify itself. Therefore, you're always eating foods that just taste good, and then clog up the body, adding more weight, making the problem more difficult, and preventing you from ever taking that weight off. I am not implying for a moment that you have to eat in such a way as to *not* enjoy your food. I'm not saying you should eat food that does not absolutely delight your taste buds. No! What I'm saying is that you can eat foods that taste fantastic but at the same time meet the requirements of your whole body.

All we're suggesting is to think in terms of eating meals that are 70 per cent high-water-content foods (fruits and vegetables) and 30 per cent concentrated foods (everything else). Wait until you see what can be done with fruits and vegetables – far more than most people imagine. The creative, innovative, and tantalizing ideas supplied in FIT FOR LIFE will probably change your eating life-style forever. When you're hungry and you think of something to eat, you're going to know about some delectable, *nonclogging* alternatives.

This can all be reduced to one simple sentence. IF YOU WANT TO BE VIBRANTLY AND VIGOROUSLY ALIVE, IN THE BEST POSSIBLE SHAPE, YOU HAVE TO EAT FOOD THAT'S ALIVE. You don't have to be a Ph.D. or a mental giant to get that. A live body will be built from live food! Food that's alive will be high-water-content food. If it does not have high water content, then that food is not alive. And if 70 per cent or more of your diet is made up of food that is dead, processed, and denatured, I leave it to you to imagine what will become of your body. Fruits and vegetables are enormously high in water. Other foods are concentrated, meaning the water has been either cooked or processed out.

Something I like to do is compare us, as a species, to the other mammals that are sharing the planet with us. Look at all the mammals. I am not talking about animals that we have as pets or in zoos, because they're under the dominion of humans and therefore have many of the problems of humans. But have you ever seen a fat tiger or impala in the wild? Have you ever seen animals in nature that have lost their teeth and use false teeth to eat, or have hearing aids to hear, or have glasses so they can see, or are wearing toupeés because they went bald, or have pacemakers to make their hearts pump, or dialysis machines for their kidneys? Have you ever heard of a million animals a year dying of heart disease? Or a half million dying of cancer? Or a quarter million dying of strokes? Or thousands dying of diabetes? *No!* In part this is because animals in the wild survive *only* by eating well and staying fit. Otherwise the process of survival of the fittest would kill them off. But for the most part, animals in nature are magnificently healthy in comparison to the health that we humans experience. And they are not overweight! Now, why is that?

All we have to do to understand this is look at the foods we are eating and look at the foods that the other mammals are eating. Other mammals, the ones living in nature, are eating live foods very high in water content. They're not eating foods that have had the water cooked or processed out. That is why they are experiencing a state of physical health much superior to ours. Even animals that are exclusively carnivorous, who eat nothing but meat, are eating high-water-content food. If you have ever had the opportunity, either in person or on film, to see a lion take down a zebra or wildebeest, you will have noticed that invariably the lion will rip open the underside of its prey, open its belly up, and go straight in and eat the intestines. I know that doesn't sound like a day at the beach, but that's how it is in the jungle! Why is it that when the lion takes down the zebra, it goes straight for the intestines? Because, by and large, carnivorous animals don't eat other carnivorous animals. Think about it: Lions don't eat tigers. Bears don't eat wolves.

Carnivorous animals are eating animals that are plant- and fruit-eaters, because that is what *all* animals need. They have to have the food from the plant kingdom. Either an animal will take its food directly from the plant kingdom, or it will eat animals that are eating that food. The reason a lion will go straight to the intestines is that there it finds the predigested high-water-content food. Then it will eat all the organs, because they have a very high water content. Then it will lap up the blood, because blood is over 90 per cent water! In other words, it goes from the inside to the outside. What is left at last is the muscle meat.

So, what we should do is make sure that a good part of the time we are eating an adequate amount of high-water-content living food. Once in a while your day's food intake won't be perfectly balanced, with 70 per cent water-content food and 30 per cent concentrated food. That's okay! We're not trying to give you some kind of jail sentence, like a diet. Once in a while concentrated food may predominate. Don't feel guilty! There is nothing to feel guilty about. You have certain cravings that you have built up over the years. It's going to take a certain amount of time for you to overcome these cravings. The idea is not to upset the balance more often than you maintain it. You eat heavy one day, and then the next day comes. It's a brand-new day. Considering that high-water-content food did not predominate the day before, the next day you should see to it that high-water-content foods *do* predominate. What is crucial, no matter what, is to keep in mind the importance of having this food high in water content on a regular basis. If it is absolutely ignored as if it made no difference, you will never be able to lose the weight that you're looking to lose and keep that weight off.

The importance of eating in this fashion can be illustrated by the words of a gentleman who has been studying these principles for over half a century. Dr Norman W. Walker is over one hundred years old.[1] He lives in Arizona. He grows his own vegetables and is still writing books. No one is pushing him around in a wheelchair or feeding him mashed bananas. He is completely independent. What is the key to his superior health and longevity? In his most recent book, *Natural Weight Control,* Dr Walker stated, 'Every plant, vegetable, fruit, nut, and seed in its raw natural state is composed of atoms and molecules. Within these atoms and molecules reside the vital elements we know as enzymes. Enzymes are not things or substances! They are the life-principle in the atoms and molecules of every living cell.

'The enzymes in the cells of the human body are exactly like those in vegetation, and the atoms in the human body each have a corresponding affinity for like atoms in vegetation. Consequently, when certain atoms are needed to rebuild or replace body cells, there will come into play a magneticlike attraction which will draw to such cells in our bodies the exact kind and type of atomic elements from the raw foods we eat.

'Accordingly, every cell in the structure of our bodies and every cell in nature's foods are infused and animated with the silent life known as enzymes. *This magneticlike attraction, however, is only available in live molecules!* (Italics mine.) Enzymes are sensitive to all heat above 130 degrees F. At 130 degrees F. they are dead. Any food which has been cooked at a temperature higher than 130 degrees F. has been subjected to the death sentence of its enzymes, and is nothing but dead food.

[1] Since the publication of this book, Dr Walker passed away, quietly, disease-free, pain-free and peacefully in his sleep of natural causes at age 109.

'Naturally, dead matter cannot do the work of live organisms. Consequently, food which has been subjected to higher temperatures above 130 degrees F. has lost its live, nutritional value. While such food can, and does, sustain life in the human system, it does so at the expense of progressively degenerating health, energy, and vitality.'

In this book and every other book Dr Walker has authored, he strongly emphasizes the importance of consuming high-water-content food if a slim, vibrant body is one of your goals. SUCCESS LEAVES CLUES! He lived to the age of 109, actively and healthfully. I would listen to him.

In 1980 the *Los Angeles Times* and *Weekly World News* carried articles about a man living in China named Wu Yunqing. Mr Yunqing is one hundred and forty-two years old and is shown riding his bicycle! When queried about his diet, he answered, 'I eat corn, rice, sweet potatoes, and other fruits and vegetables.' SUCCESS LEAVES CLUES!

In January 1973 *National Geographic* had a story by a scientist named Alexander Leaf. Dr Leaf went in search of the oldest people in the world. He found the three most consistently long-lived people to be the Abkhazians of Russia, the Vilcabambans of Ecuador, and the Hunzukuts of Pakistan. Aside from finding *no obesity* whatsoever among the Vilcabambans and Hunzukuts and very little amongst the Abkhazians, he discovered that these people were amazingly disease-free. *No* cancer! *No* heart disease! Plus most of them were living to be over one hundred years old and remaining very physically active. Dr Leaf's inquiries into these people's dietary habits indicate that the Abkhazians eat approximately 70 per cent high-water-content food and the Vilcabambans and Hunzukuts eat over 80 per cent. He and many gerontologists were stunned to learn of these people and their magnificent longevity. But, I tell you, **SUCCESS LEAVES CLUES!**

If you have written down a list of everything you ate in one day, please take it out and look at it now. I have two questions for you. First, is what you consumed about 70 per cent high-water-content food (fresh fruits and vegetables and their juices)? And second, is it a typical day's fare? If the list does not reflect 70 per cent high-water-content food and it *is* a typical day, then that list represents the *major contributing factor* to your weight problem. Not that other factors in one's life don't contribute to a weight problem; they do. Stress, psychological factors, one's job, emotions, all contribute. But all the other factors combined don't equal the influence that food has on one's weight. The old cliché 'An apple a day keeps the doctor away' was certainly on the right track. It should be 'An apple (an orange, and a few other pieces of fruit) and a salad a day will keep the doctor away.' A bit more cumbersome to state, but right on the money.

Before continuing, let's answer the common question 'What about drinking water? I drink eight glasses a day, and should I do that or should I not do that?' Actually, as you eat more foods that contain a lot of water, you will not have as much of a desire or requirement for water. In other words, people who are drinking eight glasses of water a day are doing so because they're not getting the water they need out of the foods that they're eating. Their diets are predominated by concentrated foods, so their bodies are continuously crying out for water, and they experience continuous thirst. You will find that you will have much less thirst if you are eating high-water-content food rather than eating foods devoid of water and then drinking the water separately. However, if you wish to drink water, you should drink distilled water if it is available. Mountain-spring water is not ideal for the human body, because it contains inorganic minerals that the human body can neither use nor precipitate out. These inorganic minerals tend to hook up with cholesterol in the system and form a thick plaque in the arteries. Distilled water does not have this effect. When you eat a piece of fruit or a vegetable, you are consuming distilled water. The minerals are taken from the soil, the plant distills them, and then you consume them. You may have heard that distilled water leaches minerals from the body. That is partially true. The minerals that are leached by distilled water are the inorganic minerals that the body cannot use. The effect, therefore, is healthful. Distilled water will not leach organic minerals that have become part of the structure of the cell system. Once a mineral has become part of the cell structure, it cannot be leached.

One more comment about water, and this is important. It is very debilitating to drink water *with* a meal. Many people eat and drink water at the same time. That is not a good practice, because there are digestive juices in the stomach that are breaking down food. If you drink water along with your meal, you dilute those juices, preventing the meal from being properly digested. *This also greatly hinders both the appropriation and the assimilation cycles, which in turn negatively affect the all-important elimination cycle while wasting a great deal of energy.*

In summary, by consuming high-water-content food, you will, in effect, wash the toxic waste from your body, thereby decreasing your weight. By continuing to eat high-water-content food, you will not allow the toxic waste to build up, and you will not put weight back on. We've made it apparent just how important the elimination cycle is in weight loss. **NO PRACTICE WILL EXPEDITE THE ELIMINATION CYCLE MORE THAN THE REGULAR**

CONSUMPTION OF AN ADEQUATE AMOUNT OF HIGH-WATER-CONTENT FOOD. It's the easiest thing in the world to verify, and you will be doing just that when you begin the program.

As important as high-water-content food is the second tool to assist you in the detoxification of your body. It is an intriguing and fascinating phenomenon known as . . .

CHAPTER 6

The Principle of Proper Food Combining

Perhaps you may have already come into contact with proper food combining. It is becoming more and more popular (and justifiably so). The importance of proper food combining has been proved as a result of intense research time and time again over the last eighty-five years. In fact, one of the first people who studied this subject is probably familiar to you. Does the name Ivan Pavlov ring a bell? In addition to his experiments on conditioned reflexes, Pavlov also did a great deal of study of proper food combining, and in 1902 he published a book entitled *The Work of the Digestive Glands*, wherein he revealed the basic fundamentals of proper food combining. Proper food combining works, and it works beautifully. There have been many studies done substantiating its value, most notably by Dr Herbert M. Shelton, who from 1928 to 1981 had a school in San Antonio, Texas, where he compiled the most extensive research data available on the proper combinations of foods.

Dr Shelton's work, backed up as long ago as 1924 in the *Journal of the American Medical Association* by

Dr Philip Norman, shows the effectiveness and validity of food combining as a science. If it is violated, a host of problems result, which are an enormous hindrance to the successful loss of weight. It stands to reason that if the appropriation cycle is encumbered in any way, then the cycles following will also suffer. **NOTHING STREAMLINES THE APPROPRIATION CYCLE MORE THAN ADHERING TO THE PRINCIPLES OF PROPER FOOD COMBINING.**

How does proper food combining fit in with the loss of excess weight? How do you start your day? Do you jump out of bed with an incredible feeling of vitality, ready to charge into the day? Or do you drag yourself out of bed and gulp down some coffee to get the day going? Do you go through your day with a positive feeling of anticipation? Or are you thinking, Gee, I hope I can make it until Friday. At the end of the day are you still full of energy? Are you looking forward to spending some time with your kids, your spouse, or your friends? Or, come evening, do you barely have enough energy to get dinner down and then collapse on the couch in front of the TV prior to passing out? The difference between these two types of days boils down to one crucial element: energy!

There's probably not a person reading this page right now who would not like to have more energy. It's like money. If I were to hand you a 50-dollar bill, would you tear it up and throw it into the street? I doubt it. If you would not take a 50-dollar bill and throw it away, would you do that to something far more important than money, your *energy*? You wouldn't knowingly, but *unknowingly* you may be doing that regularly. If you want to run, read, play, or do anything, you require energy. In fact if there is *no* energy in your body, it means that you are not alive. No energy, no life.

Everyone wants to have *more* energy. Guess what

function of the human body demands more energy than any other function? *The digestion of food!* Isn't that interesting? Have you ever felt sleepy after a meal? Who hasn't? That happens because all energies are concentrated on taking care of the food in the system. The digestion of food takes more energy than running, swimming, or bike riding. In fact, there's nothing you can name that takes *more* energy than the digestion of food.

This energy is crucial for the all-important detoxification (elimination of toxic waste) of the body. If we can eliminate toxic waste from our bodies on a regular basis, we are going to lose weight on a regular basis, and *not* put that weight back on. It takes energy to eliminate, and the elimination cycle is of extreme importance. The body cannot eliminate toxic waste without your cooperation. The way we must assist the body is to supply it with readily available energy on a steady basis. This is the answer to being healthy and trim. It's having a sufficient amount of energy at the body's disposal to take care of detoxification. If the digestion of food takes more energy than any other function of the body, where is it, do you think, that we are most likely to be able to free up some energy for use elsewhere? From our digestive tracts, of course.

Food combining is based on the discovery that certain combinations of food may be digested with greater ease and efficiency than others. The successful results obtained through the principles of food combining can be explained and substantiated by the facts of physiological chemistry, particularly the chemistry of digestion. Energy is the key, and nothing streamlines the process of digestion, which *optimizes* energy, more than proper food combining.

Food combining teaches this: **THE HUMAN BODY IS NOT DESIGNED TO DIGEST MORE THAN ONE CONCENTRATED FOOD IN**

THE STOMACH AT THE SAME TIME. This is a very simple but significant statement. Remember what is meant by concentrated food: ANY FOOD THAT IS NOT A FRUIT AND IS NOT A VEGETABLE IS CONCENTRATED. Proper food combining merely states that because the human stomach is not capable of digesting more than one of these concentrated foods at a time, you should not eat more than one concentrated food at a time. It's just that simple.

Every species of mammal has a specific type of digestive system biologically adapted to a particular type of food – from the lion, whose digestive tract is about twelve feet long, to the giraffe, whose digestive tract is about two hundred and eighty feet long! There are carnivorous, herbivorous, omnivorous, graminivorous and frugivorous animals on this planet. There is some argument as to what type of digestive system the human species possesses, but one thing is certain: Humans do *not* possess ALL these different types of digestive systems. However, we humans eat the diet of a lion, a giraffe, a pig, a horse, and an ape. And not only do we eat the different diets of all these animals, but we do so at the same meal! This places a tremendous burden on the digestive faculties, forces the creation of toxic waste in the system, and squanders a great deal of precious energy.

I wonder if you have ever eaten meat and potatoes together. Fish and rice? Chicken and noodles? Eggs and toast? Cheese and bread? Cereal and milk? You might be saying, 'Hey, wait a second here, what else is left?' Don't worry, there's plenty. What if I were to tell you that eating these particular combinations is *not* in your best interest and also insures that you will have neither the slim body *nor* the energy you want? In fact, regularly eating these particular combinations *guarantees* that you will never have the energy that you need.

The cornerstone of weight loss is detoxification, and detoxification is entirely dependent upon energy. The improper combination of food in the stomach is exactly why we have an 'energy crisis' in this country. It is also a contributing factor to why people in this country are dying at age 50. Death means the body no longer has the energy to deal with its situation. And death at 50 is indefensible.

Nearly two thirds of the population are overweight. A great deal of that can be attributed to the fact that we eat foods haphazardly and indiscriminately combined. This deserves further explanation. Let's use meat and potatoes, because that is something that probably everyone has eaten at one time or another. Even though I am talking about meat and potatoes, I could easily be talking about fish and rice, or chicken and noodles, or bread and cheese. Consider eating a steak. You prepare it the way you like it and then you eat it. Once in the stomach, this concentrated protein requires a particular digestive juice to break it down – an acid juice. At the same time you're going to have a baked potato.

Now, you might be saying, 'Wait a minute, potato – that's a vegetable.' True, potato is a vegetable. If you were to bite into a *raw* potato and chew it up, it would be a high-water-content food in your stomach. But once it is baked, you can chew it until your jaw atrophies and it will not turn to water. Once it is baked, most of the water has been removed and it is of a very concentrated, starchy nature. So this concentrated starch enters the stomach with the steak. The digestive juice necessary to break this food down is not acid, but alkaline. If you have ever taken a chemistry class, you will know what happens when acid and alkaline come into contact with each other. They neutralize each other.

So you have just eaten a steak and potato. They've gone into your stomach, and the digestive juices necessary to break them down have just been neutralized. What is going to happen to that food? The body, which is infinitely wise, immediately recognizes an emergency, because a number-one priority for the body is the digestion of food. The body is literally thrown into turmoil. It has to secrete more digestive juices. This takes time and energy. New digestive juices are secreted into the stomach, and what happens? They are neutralized again. Now the body is really pushed to its limit. More energy is needed to secrete even *more* juices into the stomach. A long time is elapsing during this process. As a matter of fact, several hours are going by as the body is manufacturing all this digestive juice. Digestive juices are secreted into the stomach once again, and we begin to experience indigestion or heartburn. Finally the food, which has never been properly digested, is simply moved out of the stomach by the peristaltic action of the intestines. This undigested food is forced into the intestines after several hours of being held up in the stomach. As if the stomach were saying, 'Here, you take it for a while!'

Exactly what has just occurred is important to understand. Most of the protein, being in the stomach for so long, has putrefied. Most of the carbohydrate has fermented. Putrefaction and fermentation are two elements the human body, under no circumstances, can use. Nutrients affected in this way cannot be incorporated into *healthy* cell structure. Foods that have been putrefied or fermented generate toxic acids in the body. Because of the putrefaction and fermentation, there is gas, flatulence, more heartburn, acid indigestion, and R-O-L-A-I-D-S. If not Rolaids, then Tums, Gelusil, Pepto-Bismol, Alka-Seltzer, Bromo Seltzer, Mylanta, or milk of magnesia. The list goes on. We take antacids by the trainload in this country. Why? Because we are eating foods haphazardly and indiscriminately.

When they are all thrown together in the stomach, the body cannot handle them. We're the only species in the world that, when finished eating, must medicate itself to move the food out of our guts.

Because there's all this putrefaction, fermentation, and resulting acid, what actually is in the stomach at that time is a mass of spoiled, rotting, foul-smelling food. Now, I know that doesn't sound too appealing, and I don't want to be rude, but I do want to be *real* – and that is exactly what is happening inside the system. The food is forced to stay in the stomach, not being digested, and it is literally rotting. The nutrients that may have existed within that food are lost. It is in the stomach for a long time, while the body uses up an incredible amount of energy. Then the food is forced into the intestines, where it travels through some thirty feet of intestinal tract. Visualize it! Thirty feet of intestines are being forced to cope with this rotten food. That is why people are tired after a meal like this. That is why people have no energy. That food may take eight hours just to get out of the stomach and twenty to forty more to get through the intestines.

In *The Hygienic System, Vol. II,* Herbert M. Shelton describes the work of Arthur Cason, M.D. Dr Cason reported in 1945 that he and his aides conducted two groups of experiments that showed that eating protein and carbohydrates at the same meal retards and even prevents digestion. He made control tests in which digestive rates were recorded and a final analysis of the feces was made. He said, 'Such tests always reveal that the digestion of proteins when mixed with starches is retarded in the stomach; the degree varying in different individuals, and also in the particular protein or starch ingested. An examination of the fecal matter reveals both undigested starch granules and protein shred and fibers, whereas, when ingested separately, each goes to a conclusion.' If food is properly combined, it is fully broken down, absorbed, and utilized by the body. No undigested fragments will show in the feces.

We also find when foods are eaten in incompatible combinations and fermentation results that alcohol is produced in the digestive tract, with the same consequences that would come from drinking alcohol and with the same potential for liver damage.

The principle of proper food combining suggests only this: We don't want to waste energy. We don't want food to sit around rotting in the stomach for eight hours and fouling up the intestines for twenty hours more. What we really want is food going into the stomach and being there approximately *three* hours with *no* putrefaction, *no* fermentation, *no* gas, *no* flatulence, *no* heartburn, and *no* acid indigestion requiring medication. We want food to pass quickly and efficiently through the intestines. The way to insure that is to have *one* concentrated food at a time, not two. Eating two concentrated foods simultaneously will cause the food to rot, and rotten food **CANNOT BE ASSIMILATED**! Improper food combining drastically thwarts the assimilation and the elimination cycles.

There is a simple way to avoid this entire problem. If you want to have a steak, or a piece of fish or chicken, so be it. Just be aware that if you're going to have any flesh food, that is your one concentrated food for *that* meal. That means with it you should not have any other concentrated foods. Not potatoes, rice, noodles, cheese, or bread, but with it have high-water-content food. In other words, along with the steak have some vegetables, say, for example, some broccoli and zucchini. It can be any vegetable that you like. Understand that vegetables do not need their own specific digestive juices. They will break down in either medium, acid or alkaline. Let's say you lightly steam some broccoli and zucchini, or stir-fry them, or sauté them, however you like your vegetables prepared. (Keep in mind that the more you cook them, the more life and water content you cook out of them.) You prepare the vegetables, and along with the steak and vegetables you have a tossed salad. Now you're not going to go hungry eating like that, are you? Of course not.

We're not suggesting that you starve yourself. What we're talking about is this: There are certain physiological limitations that the human body has, and they have to be respected, that's all. If you want to have the baked potato, great! Have a baked potato. Have it with some butter, preferably raw butter if available. And with it have the vegetables: zucchini, string beans, broccoli, whatever you like, and your salad. Again, you do not have to go hungry. Can you see what food combining suggests? You want to have meat? Have meat with vegetables and salad. You want to have potatoes? Have potatoes with vegetables and salad. You want to have bread? Have bread with vegetables and salad. You want to have pasta? Have pasta with garlic butter and vegetables and salad. You want to have cheese? Take the cheese and chop it and put it in your salad, *without croutons.* Or melt cheese on your vegetables. This may sound overly simple to people who fear they will not get enough protein unless they eat meat at every meal – but I'll address that subject in Chapter 7.

You see, you're enjoying yourself when you eat, you're eating the foods you like, but you're not throwing them all together and eating them all at the same time. This practice not only optimizes the extraction and utilization of nutrients in the food (because there is no putrefaction or fermentation), but also puts an end to painful digestive disorders and substantially increases available energy. Violation of proper food combining has many negative consequences, and many positive results come from adhering to its principles. Let's go for the positive! **POSITIVE NUMBER ONE: WEIGHT LOSS!**

It is occasionally argued that nature itself combines starches and proteins in the same food, and if nature does, we may do so also. This objection is not valid. If a food that is a *natural* protein-starch combination (such as beans) is eaten alone, the body is capable of modifying its digestive juices and timing their secretions in such ways that digestion can go on with a fair degree of efficiency.[1] But when a separate starch food and a separate protein food are eaten at the same meal, this precise adaption of the digestive secretions to the character and digestive requirements of the food is not possible. There is a marked and important difference between eating a food that is a natural protein-starch combination and eating two foods, one a protein and the other a starch.

If it's not good to mix a protein and a starch, is it okay to mix a protein with another protein or a starch with a starch? Actually, the most ideal situation is **ONE** concentrated food per meal, so that would preclude mixing protein with protein or starch with starch. However, one of these combinations is acceptable: a starch with a starch. The reason that two proteins should not be mixed is that proteins are of such different character and complex composition that the modifications necessary to meet the digestive requirements of more than one protein food are impossible. Therefore, both proteins putrefy in the system. This does not mean that two different kinds of flesh may not be eaten together or that two different kinds of nuts may

[1] We say *fair* because beans are notoriously difficult to digest. Most people after eating beans will experience gas and flatulence, proving the point that protein-starch combinations of *any* kind cause problems.

not be eaten together; but it certainly means that no two *different* proteins – flesh, eggs, dairy products or nuts – should be eaten simultaneously.

Starches are not as difficult to break down as protein, so more than one starch can be eaten together. For example, if you wanted to have croutons on a salad and also wanted to have a baked potato, it would work digestively without fermentation. Rice and beans, although heavy, is another combination that can be compatible in the stomach. Or if you were having an avocado sandwich and wanted to have some corn chips with it, that would work as well. Of course, to reiterate, only one of these foods at a time would be *best,* because it would mean less work for the body, resulting in less energy expenditure. But two starches *can* be combined without spoiling in the stomach.

By introducing you to proper food combining we're suggesting that you start to alter some of your existing dietary habits. It is not something that has to turn your life upside down at all. It's something to be done as much as possible *at your own pace!* Of course, the more you practice it, the more success you will have. The more frequently it is done, the more quickly you are going to be able to lose the weight you're looking to lose. Can you see how simple this information is? What we're talking about here is a new way of eating. It's obvious that we need it! The way we have been eating in this country for the last hundred years or so has brought us to the point where *over half* of us are struggling with weight problems. We have never been taught the proper way to nourish the body. Obviously, from what we have just learned, the standard approach to nutrition – the four-food-group philosophy – does not work. It is an archaic, counterproductive approach to eating. I know that the four-food-group philosophy has been nutritional gospel for many years, but the evidence against it is staring us in the face. It has not worked, evidenced by the fact that so many people in this country are sick and overweight. And the problem is far from under control. At a recent conference on obesity at the Johns Hopkins University School of Medicine, attended by researchers and clinicians who deal with obesity, Dr Gerard Smith of Cornell University Medical Center, addressing himself to the physiological cues that turn feeding behavior on and off, said, 'We don't know where to look and haven't found the cues. The extent of our ignorance is total.' The lunch served at this gathering consisted of roast beef with mashed potatoes and gravy, broccoli, Jell-O, and chocolate pie. Their ignorance of the principles of proper food combining is most assuredly total. Were it not for the time-honored belief in the four-food-group approach to eating, such grievous food combinations would not be so commonplace.

For some, forsaking the four-food-group myth may be hard. But the only thing that makes it hard is the belief system people have built over the years. Belief systems *can* be the biggest obstacle to one's progress. If the belief in something is strong enough, no amount of evidence or proof of its falsity can dissuade the believer. Consider the plight of Galileo three centuries ago, severely chastised for his ridiculous belief that the sun did not orbit the earth. Galileo, whose theory was based on Copernicus's earlier work, was sent to jail for insinuating something as preposterous as the sun not orbiting the earth. Why, any fool could go outside in the morning and *watch* the sun as it traveled across the sky, plopping into the ocean or disappearing behind a mountain every night. Right? Wrong! I daresay that no one today believes that the sun circles the earth. But it sure looks that way, doesn't it? It's the same thing with certain dietary habits we have. They look as if they're right, but they're exactly wrong! Over three hundred years after Galileo's observations were made public, and even though he was right and everyone else was wrong, the Catholic Church is just getting around to exonerating him for being right! Traditions, no matter how fallacious they may be, die hard.

Proper food combining does not prevent you from eating the foods you like; you just shouldn't eat them all at the same time. If you eat in accordance with the principle of compatibily combining foods, there will be no enormous loss of energy. *There will be an energy surplus.* Do you remember when you had your last Thanksgiving meal? After eating, did you happen to utter that famous sentence, 'Uhh! I'll never eat again'? Many of us have used it. After the meal, you go to the living room and sit down and that's it. 'I'm just going to watch the rest of the game. A cup of coffee? Okay. Huh, a piece of pie? Well, okay.' You can't even bend over! You have to slide into the chair. Well, why? Because you had so many combinations of foods. You had the turkey, and I'm not saying not to have turkey on Thanksgiving, but along with the turkey, there was probably a roast beef or a ham, or *both.* You had a little of each. Then there are the mashed potatoes and yams. You had some of those. And the stuffing! Of course, you had to have the stuffing, *with* gravy. And those biscuits, and pumpkin pie. And a token vegetable on the side that nobody touches. You know what I'm talking about? I'm not suggesting that you not participate in Thanksgiving. But the reason the body is totally exhausted after a meal like that is that there are so many different, concentrated, incompatible foods in the stomach at one time, the system is thrown into turmoil. Doing this once in a while, the body has a chance to deal with the situation. On a regular basis, however, the body breaks down. After nourishing the body, especially at a celebration, we should feel vibrant and ready to conquer the world. Instead, we're barely able to conquer the couch.

Do you remember the lion that we were talking about before, that took down the zebra? When that lion ate the zebra, it wasn't having baked potato with it. It's strictly à la carte out there in the jungle. The animals in nature experience a much higher level of health than we do; not only eating high-water-content food, they are also properly combining their food. *Animals in nature don't combine their foods improperly.* That is the beauty of it. They eat one food at a time. Not like us. We eat anything we can get our hands on, including them!

Here's something that may surprise you: Henry Ford was also a proponent of food combining. In an article from *Early American Life,* David L. Lewis discusses the 'Wayside Inn,' a vocational school set up by Ford in 1928 to 'teach boys how to work with their hands and how to think.' Underprivileged boys between the ages of twelve and seventeen were enrolled in the ninth through twelfth grades. They received training in agriculture, electrical and automotive engineering, plumbing, carpentry, and other vocations as well as academic subjects. 'Along with a Ford-financed education, the students had to suffer Ford's theory on diet. Sugar, candy, cakes, pies, puddings, and other kinds of sweet desserts were forbidden, as well as tea, cocoa, and table salts. **STARCHES AND PROTEINS WERE NEVER MIXED BECAUSE THEY WERE CONSIDERED TO BE CHEMICALLY INCOMPATIBLE** [emphasis mine], while vegetable salads were served twice a day.' All right, Henry! He wasn't about to feed them ill-combined meals; they wouldn't have any energy left for work!

It is essential that we start to respect our digestive limitations. We need to free up energy to get toxic waste out of our bodies. The digestive tract uses more energy than any other function of the body. Food combining frees up that energy so your body can work to detoxify itself. And the beautiful thing *is you don't have to go hungry.* How would you like to be 10 pounds lighter 10 days from now, *while eating?* Well, of course, anyone who is overweight would like to do that. Just by making use of your new understanding of proper food combining, it is possible for you to achieve that. Food combining works! This is not something that you have to take my word for. All you have to do is start to combine your foods the way I have described, and you will know exactly whether or not this information is true. That, after all, is what really counts, isn't it? *Does it work?* Whether it is proved or not proved means nothing. If you can dramatically increase your energy, do away with stomach ailments, lose weight, and feel good by properly combining, would it matter to you if it was 'proved' not to work? Of course not. Don't believe me. Try it!

Proper food combining simply creates the environment for weight loss. If you can eat food and have it go through your stomach in three hours instead of eight, there are five hours of energy right there that you have picked up – five hours to be put toward detoxification and weight loss. And you're going to pick up more energy as that food goes through the intestines with great ease.

Some people have said to me, 'This makes pretty much sense, I have to admit, but I'm a businessman, I go out for lunch every day, so I can't do this.' Why not? You can adhere to this principle in any restaurant you wish. Any good restaurant will allow you to order what you want. You are the customer. You are paying. You can have what you want. You can go in with your business associates and say, 'What is today's special?'

'Today we have fresh trout, absolutely fantastic.'

'Wonderful! I'll have the trout, and instead of the rice that comes with the trout, what vegetables do you have this afternoon?'

'Well, we have fresh asparagus and cauliflower.'

'Fantastic! I'll have the trout and vegetables, and would you please bring me a salad with that?'

You're going to be able to participate in ordering and eat your lunch, and your business associates are not going to say, 'Hey, how come you're not eating the rice?' No one's going to say anything. The beautiful thing is that when you and your business associates stand up, you are going to feel light and be able to finish the rest of your day with abundant energy, and your business associates are going to have stomachs full of rotting food that will hold them back. They'll feel tired and will have to pick themselves up with coffee or some other toxic, addictive stimulant. What's so fantastic about proper food combining is that it dramatically improves your level of energy and at the same time it frees up everything necessary within the body to rid itself of the excess toxic waste that is keeping you heavy.

I know it sounds simple, and the marvelous thing abut this method is that it *is* simple! You just make little changes. If it took you twenty, or thirty, or forty years to build up the problem, you have plenty of time to turn it around, but the important thing is *you have to start.* I get excited and carried away each time I discuss this subject, because I know how simple and obvious this information is. I have seen it work with thousands of people, and I know that thousands of other people, including you, can start to experience this wonderful feeling of control, of knowing how to have a trim body, and then doing what is necessary to make that body appear. It's within your grasp – yours for the asking.

By the way, the people of the United States spend

some thirty billion dollars on drugs every year. They swallow 25 million pills every hour! Do you know what the number-one-selling prescription drug in the United States is? It used to be Valium. According to the *Wall Street Journal,* it is now Tagamet. And what is Tagamet for? *Stomach disorders!* Could that possibly have anything to do with what people's stomachs are forced to deal with every day?

As you start to experiment with the proper combinations of food, you will come to realize firsthand what a truly marvelous tool proper food combining is in the quest to lose weight. (Refer to the back of this book to find out how to obtain the FIT FOR LIFE Proper Food Combining Chart.)

This brings us now to the third tool designed to remove toxic waste from your body. It is the one I enjoy discussing more than any other, since it revolves around . . .

CHAPTER 7

The Principle of Correct Fruit Consumption

In the broad subject of health there is surely no area that has been more misunderstood, more unjustly maligned, or more abused than the consumption of fruit. People do not know how to eat fruit in this country. I don't mean that they don't know how to pick it up and eat it; they have that down pat. I mean that they don't know *when* or *how* to eat it. The correct consumption of fruit is very closely associated with proper food combining.

How many people do you know who truly detest fruit? Who really can't stand it? Probably none. Most of the people you will ever talk to will readily express their fondness of fruit. About the most negative comment you will ever hear about fruit is 'I love it, but it doesn't love me.' Or 'I love it, but I can't eat it.' Why they can't eat it and why they have to be careful with it is more often than not based on some misunderstanding about the nature of correct fruit consumption.

At every seminar I have ever given, I ask for a show of hands from those who dislike fruit, and rarely, even in groups of seven hundred people or more, does even one hand go up. The reason almost everyone expresses a liking for fruit is that our bodies crave it *instinctively*. With its sweet blends of rare flavors, delightful aromas, and eye-pleasing colors, fruit is always an invitation to pleasure in eating. Fruit is, without doubt, the most beneficial, energy-giving, life-enhancing food you can eat. IF! If it is correctly consumed. What you are about to learn may be met with a certain amount of skepticism, as it attacks your belief system about fruit, and that's all right. It involves a new way of thinking about your body and how you nourish it.

Young and old alike think of fruit as a treat. A cold piece of melon on a hot day – delicious! You eat a spicy meal and eat a piece of fruit, and it cools and soothes the palate.

This may surprise you: The reason we instinctively crave fruit is that fruit, without any question, is the most important food we can put into the human body. It is the one food that the human species is biologically adapted to.

On 15 May 1979, *The New York Times* ran a story on the work of Dr Alan Walker, an eminent anthropologist at John Hopkins University. The story was a bombshell for those doctors, dietitians, and nutritionists not aware of the immense importance of fruit in the human diet. Dr Walker's findings indicate that our 'early human ancestors were not predominantly meat eaters or even eaters of seeds, shoots, leaves or grasses. Nor were they omnivorous. Instead, they appear to have subsisted chiefly on a diet of fruit.' Dr Walker developed a fascinating way of determining dietary trends by studying striations, or markings, on teeth. All foods leave distinctly different markings on teeth. In his studies of fossilized teeth Dr Walker noted that, to date, 'No exceptions have been found. Every tooth examined from the hominids of the 12-million-year period leading up to Homo erectus appeared to be that of a fruit eater.' **WOW!** You can practically hear the gnashing of teeth over at the Cattlemen's Association.

Since fruit is what we are biologically adapted to eat, it is far more important for you to think in terms of how much fruit you're going to eat than how much protein you're going to get during the day. In 15 years I've never met a person with a protein deficiency, notwithstanding the fact that it does exist in devastating circumstances such as kwashiorkor. Yet I have met hundreds with protein poisoning, and most of them were not eating a sufficient amount of fruit. Overconsumption of protein has been linked to breast, liver, and bladder cancer and to an increase in the incidence of leukemia.[1] According to William J. Mayo, founder of the Mayo Clinic, in an address before the American College of Surgeons, 'Meat-eating has increased 400 per cent in the last 100 years. Cancer of the stomach forms nearly one third of all cancers of the human body. If flesh foods are not fully broken up, decompositions result, and active poisons are thrown into an organ not intended for their reception.'[2] Protein poisoning is hyperacidity in the body, which is discussed in Chapter 9.

It was stated earlier that it is imperative for the system to be constantly cleansed of the toxic waste that builds in the body. The most effective way for this cleansing to be accomplished is with the consumption of high-water-content food. You can probably surmise the next sentence. **FRUIT HAS THE HIGHEST WATER CONTENT OF ANY**

[1] Viktoras Kulvinskas. *Survival into the 21st Century*. Wethersfield, Connecticut: Omangod Press, 1975.
[2] Blanche Leonardo, Ph.D. *Cancer and Other Diseases from Meat Consumption*. Santa Monica, California: Leaves of Healing, 1979.

FOOD. All fruit is 80 per cent to 90 per cent cleansing, life-giving water. In addition, all the vitamins, minerals, carbohydrates, amino acids, and fatty acids that the human body requires for its existence are to be found in fruit. The life force inherent in fruit is unsurpassed by any other food. When fruit is *correctly* consumed, nothing can match its benefits. By its nature fruit affords the body the opportunity to cleanse built-up residue from the system. In this cleansed state every aspect of your life is enhanced. Your body is capable of functioning at its optimum efficiency.

As a tool in weight loss the proper consumption of fruit is unparalleled in its effectiveness and efficiency. In October 1983 a Yale University professor, Judith Rodin, presented some interesting data to the International Congress on Obesity in New York. Her studies of the benefits of fruit sugar indicate that 'What you eat in one meal really affects what you will eat in the next meal.' The *Bergen Record* reported that Ms. Rodin gave plain water sweetened with different kinds of sugar to a study group. 'The people who drank the liquid sweetened with the fruit sugar fructose ate significantly less than people who drank either water or liquid sweetened with the common sugar sucrose.' She and her fellow researchers noted that 'the subjects who consumed fructose ate an average of 479 calories less [at their next meal] than the people who had sucrose.'

Dr William Castelli, medical director of the famed Framingham (Massachusetts) Study on Heart Disease and a faculty member at Harvard Medical School, indicates that 'An amazing substance found in many types of fruit can cut your risk of heart disease or heart attack. The substance protects the heart by preventing the blood from becoming too thick and plugging up the arteries.' Fruit is *cleansing, not clogging.*

The ingredient essential for a vigorous life is energy. We already know that digestion uses more energy than any other physical activity. Here is where fruit performs a most vital and significant role. **FRUIT REQUIRES LESS ENERGY TO BE DIGESTED THAN ANY OTHER FOOD.** In fact, it demands practically none!

Here's why: Everything consumed by the human body must eventually be broken down and transformed into glucose, fructose, glycerine, amino acids, and fatty acids. The brain cannot function on *anything* but glucose (sugar). Fruit *is* glucose in the body. Its digestion, absorption, and assimilation require only a minute fraction of the energy necessary to break down other foods. Other foods spend anywhere from one and a half to four hours in the stomach. (And that is only if what is eaten is properly combined.) The less concentrated and the better combined the foods, the less time spent in the stomach. The more concentrated and ill-combined, the longer they spend in the stomach. The stomach is where the initial expenditure of energy takes place. **FRUIT DOES NOT DIGEST IN THE STOMACH!** Not even minimally. Fruits are predigested. All fruits (with the exception of bananas, dates, and dried fruit, which stay in the stomach a bit longer) are in the stomach only a very short time. They pass *through* the stomach in twenty to thirty minutes, as if they were going through a tunnel. They break down and release their supercharged, life-giving nutrients in the intestines.

The energy fruit conserves by not having to be broken down in the stomach is considerable. This energy is automatically redirected to cleanse the body of toxic waste, thereby reducing weight. All this is true *only* when fruit is correctly consumed, however. What constitutes correct consumption? It is actually quite simple. Since fruit is not intended to be in the stomach extensively, correct consumption means that **FRUIT**

SHOULD NEVER BE EATEN WITH OR IMMEDIATELY FOLLOWING ANYTHING. It is essential that when you eat fruit, it is eaten on an *empty* stomach. THIS IS UNQUESTIONABLY THE MOST IMPORTANT ASPECT OF FIT FOR LIFE. If you eat fruit correctly, because it has so much water and demands so little energy to digest, it will play a major role in enabling your body to detoxify your system, supplying you with a great deal of energy for weight loss and other life activities. Fruit is *the* most important food you can eat. But if fruit is eaten on top of other foods, many problems result.

Say you eat a sandwich, and then you eat a piece of fruit – for example, a piece of melon. The piece of melon is ready to go straight through the stomach into the intestines, but it is prevented from doing so. In the interim the whole meal rots and ferments and turns to acid. The very instant that fruit comes into contact with food in the stomach and digestive juices the entire mass of food begins to spoil. Whatever protein is in the stomach putrefies, whatever carbohydrate is there ferments. The whole thing turns to acid, and we run for medication because of the discomfort. This is something that is easily verifiable. Perhaps you have already experienced it.

Perhaps after a meal you have had a piece of fruit or a glass of juice, and you noticed a sharp pain in your stomach, or indigestion or heartburn. The reason for that discomfort was that you ate fruit that would have gone straight through the stomach into the intestines, but was prevented by the other food from doing so. *Medical* evidence for this process is not to be found, because the effects of diet on the body have not yet been *sufficiently* studied by the medical profession, and its practitioners are the first to admit this. However, Dr Herbert M. Shelton, *the* authority on food combining, stresses that the potential value of fruit can be realized only if it is consumed on an *empty* stomach. If you have consumed fruit improperly consistently and not felt sick, that does not mean you have not violated a dietary law. It only shows the tremendous adaptability of our bodies. You can avoid paying income taxes and appear to get away with it. That doesn't mean you haven't broken the law. Ultimately the IRS will catch up with you. Prolonged abuse of the correct-consumption-of-fruit principle will ultimately take its toll.

Many people eat melon incorrectly and then blame the discomfort on the melon. They say, 'You know, I can't eat melon. Every time I eat melon, I burp it up all night.' Well, what happened? They ate a piece of melon *after* a sandwich or some other food, and instead of passing swiftly into the intestines, it was stopped by the other food. It then fermented in the stomach and the victim burped it up all night. The melon was blamed, whereas, if the melon were eaten first and about twenty minutes were allowed to elapse, the melon would have left the stomach intact, and the other food eaten would then enter the stomach, and no problems would result.

This is a very simple tool you are being given, and most people have never even heard of this. Physiologically fruit passes through the system rapidly and does not use the huge amounts of energy demanded by other foods. This is why I say, without any hesitation whatsoever, that **FRUIT IS THE MOST IMPORTANT FOOD THAT YOU CAN POSSIBLY EAT**! This goes for **ALL** fruit, even the acid fruits such as oranges, pineapples, and grapefruits. These are only classified botanically as acid fruits. Once inside the body all fruit becomes alkaline if it is consumed correctly. In point of fact, fruit as well as vegetables have the unique ability to neutralize the acids that build in our systems. Improper food combinations, an insufficient quantity of high-water-content food, the by-products of many concentrated foods, food additives, polluted air and water, stress – all these and more cause the system to toxify and acidify. A toxic acid system can be recognized by bloating, excess weight, cellulite, graying hair, balding, nervous outbursts, dark circles under the eyes, and premature lines in the face. Ulcers are a direct result of corrosive acid in the system. Fruit, if properly eaten, has the marvelous rejuvenating capability to counteract the acids in the system. When you have totally mastered the principle of correct fruit consumption, you have tuned in to one of nature's secrets of beauty, longevity, health, energy, happiness, and normal weight.

Fruit, more than any other food, most perfectly supplies the body with what it needs to experience the highest level of health possible. Aside from its high water content for cleansing, the fact that it leaves no toxic residue in the system and that it demands hardly any energy for digestion makes it the most perfectly balanced food for supplying the prerequisites of life for your body. The five essentials of life that must come from the foods you eat are glucose for fuel (from carbohydrates), amino acids, minerals, fatty acids, and vitamins. The number-one, most important priority of any food is its fuel value. Without fuel the body cannot exist. Fuel value should always be the foremost factor in determining the worth of any food. The ideal percentage of each of the five essentials in food as required by the human body is as follows:

glucose	–	90%
amino acids	–	4%–5%
minerals	–	3%–4%
fatty acids	–	1+%
vitamins	–	under 1%

The above represents what the ideal composition of food, in terms of the body's needs, would be. There is only one food on the planet that fills that bill perfectly. It's fruit! This would support Dr Alan Walker's findings that human beings were strict frugivores for millions of years. Before we, as a race, were led astray by external influences, like all other animals in nature we *instinctively* ate what most efficiently supplied us with the prerequisites of life. In our case this was **FRUIT**.

There are two important considerations crucial to mastering the correct consumption of fruit. The first concerns what type of fruit or fruit juice to consume. There is only one type: **FRESH**! This cannot be overemphasized. There is no benefit whatsoever in eating fruit that has been processed or altered in any way by heat. There is, however, considerable detriment. The body is capable of utilizing fruit *only* in its natural state. Baked apples, any canned fruit, cooked applesauce, and fruit pies are all harmful in that they supply *no* cleansing and *no* nutrients, and they are toxic and acidic in the body, possibly damaging the sensitive linings of the inner organs. They force the body to use its precious energy to neutralize their acidity and get it out of the body. The fact is that fruit has a delicate nature. Cooking *destroys* its potential value.

There is no question that the philosophies of macrobiotics (which discourages fruit eating) and Natural Hygiene are not in agreement on this point. Over the past ten years in my private practice I have had occasion to counsel dozens of macrobiotic enthusiasts. They came to me because they were feeling unwell after prolonged adherence to the theories of macrobiotics. After several weeks on a hygienic diet, *all of them* experienced improvement in their well-being. Their marked improvement came so easily, I believe, because they had the good groundwork laid by macrobiotics, which is head and shoulders above the average American diet but at a disadvantage in its misinterpretation of the benefits of fruit, requiring that no fruit be eaten raw. That is a misconception. All fruit consumed *must* be fresh and uncooked, or the many benefits described here are lost. The same holds true for fruit juice. It must be fresh. If it has been pasteurized, as is the case with orange juice made from concentrate, it is pure acid before you even drink it. Drinking a liquid that is pure acid hampers rather than aids the quest for weight loss.

You may ask, 'Why drink juice at all, wouldn't the whole food be better?' Actually, yes. A whole food *is* always more acceptable than one that has been fragmented. However, people do like to drink something. Rather than habit-forming and toxic drinks such as coffee, tea, alcohol, sodas, and milk, it would be wiser to drink fruit *or* vegetable juices. A good point to remember is not to gulp juice down. Because it is fragmented, you should take but a mouthful at a time and let it mix with your saliva before swallowing it.

Fruit is packed, brimming over, with the vital forces of life. Correctly utilized, it can be put to the immediate service of your body. The cleansing and weight loss it occasions and the energy it saves are unequaled by any other food. To destroy all its beneficial effects by consuming it at the wrong time or in the wrong state is nothing short of a crime against your body! Could you enjoy the Mona Lisa if mud were smeared all over it? Could you appreciate the recording of a Mozart sonata if there were a deep scratch in the record? Could you delight in the scent of a rose if garbage were dumped on it? You cheat yourself of the many positive benefits of fruit if you allow it to spoil in your digestive tract.

The second consideration pertains to the amount of time that should elapse between eating foods other than fruit and then eating fruit. As long as your stomach is empty, you can eat all the fruit you wish over as long a period as you wish, *so long as twenty to thirty minutes elapse before eating anything else.* This will allow the time necessary for the fruit or juice to leave your stomach. Juice and some fruits take less time, but twenty to thirty minutes is a good standard to use to be sure. Bananas, dates, and dried fruit need about forty-five minutes to one hour. Once you have eaten *anything* other than fruit, you must wait *at least* three hours. If any flesh food is eaten, at least four hours. These times pertain *only* to foods that were eaten in accordance with proper food combining. If you should eat a meal that is not properly combined, the food will probably be in your stomach for at least eight hours. You should therefore not consume any fruit or fruit juice during that time.

HOW LONG TO WAIT AFTER EATING OTHER FOOD BEFORE YOU CAN AGAIN EAT FRUIT

FOOD	TIME TO WAIT
Salad or raw vegetables	*2 hours*
Properly combined meal, without flesh	*3 hours*
Properly combined meal, with flesh	*4 hours*
Any improperly combined meal	*8 hours*

Fruit plays an extremely important role in FIT FOR LIFE. We're not going to tell you anything outlandish, like the enzymes in certain fruits burn fat so that you feel you have permission to overeat anything you want and then burn it away with irrational quantities of fruit. That would be not only irresponsible but also a physiological absurdity. One of the foremost roles that fruit plays in FIT FOR LIFE is that of *resting* the digestive tract, thereby freeing up energy to be utilized in cleansing, repair, and weight loss.

Obviously, proper food combining and the correct consumption of fruit deal extensively with not only *what* you eat but also *when.*

If someone were to ask you what you thought was the worst time of day to eat, I wonder what you would say. Probably 'Right before going to sleep,' as so many other people think. Even though eating right before going to sleep is a horrible habit, it's second to the most counterproductive and destructive time of day to eat. And that time is in the morning when you awake. WHAT? I can hear your shrieks of disbelief from here. 'But what about all those admonitions about having a hearty breakfast for energy?' What about them? Do you know what the all-American coffee break is in this country? People eat a big, hearty breakfast 'for energy,' and the body is so tired from the work of digesting it that 'pick-me-ups' are the only way people can make it through to lunch without falling asleep! I know what a tremendous blow this is to one of the most conditioned and deep-rooted belief systems.

Just for a moment try to forget everything you thought was true about breakfast. Try to forget for a moment all the advice of the nutritionists, dietitians, doctors, and other experts. Just for a moment rely only on your own common sense for an answer as to whether breakfast has a positive or negative influence on your weight.

Remember, ENERGY IS THE ESSENCE OF LIFE. When you wake up in the morning, you are rested and at the height of your energy level for the day, provided that your system did not spend the night contending with a 'midnight snack' or miscombined meal. On what are you going to expend that morning burst of energy? A 'hearty breakfast'? You know that digestion uses an enormous amount of energy. A hearty breakfast, which is usually a slap in the face of the principles of proper food combining, cannot *bring* you energy! IT USES IT! How else could the food be digested if energy were not being expended? Most traditional breakfasts of toast and eggs, or cereal with milk, or meat and potatoes are ill-combined, forcing the body to work for hours *spending* its energy. Food spends approximately three hours or more in the stomach alone if properly combined. Energy can't even start to be built until food is absorbed from the intestines. Strictly from the standpoint of energy, does it make sense to have breakfast when you wake up in the morning? If breakfast is skipped, not only will you *not* pass out from lack of food (your body is actually still using the food eaten the day before), but you will be far more alert and energetic.

The word *breakfast* is actually a distortion of the words *break* and *fast*. Originally the word *breakfast* was used to indicate the meal used to break a fast. A fast is the abstention from food for an extended length of time, not one night's sleep.

An integral part of **FIT FOR LIFE** is this: **FROM THE TIME YOU WAKE UP IN THE MORNING UNTIL AT LEAST NOON, CONSUME NOTHING BUT FRESH FRUIT AND FRUIT JUICE**. Eat or drink as much as you desire; put no limitations on how much you want. If you desire it, have it; but listen to your body – don't overeat! If you have nothing but fruit and fruit juice, you will be able to create, not burn up, a huge chunk of your available energy for the day. Fruit demands practically no energy to be digested, because it does not digest in the stomach. It needs no further digestion if well chewed.

The intestines are where all nutrients are absorbed.

Because fruit finds its way into the intestines within minutes instead of hours, its nutrients are immediately absorbed and utilized by the body. By eating fruit you make your entire day more productive and more energetic, because you have conserved rather than squandered your energy. You will be amazed at what an incredibly dramatic effect this will have on your entire life once you adjust to **ONLY FRUIT AND FRUIT JUICES UNTIL NOON**. After experiencing the wonderful benefits, you will wonder why you ever ate a heavy meal first thing in the morning. A heavy breakfast means a heavy day. A light breakfast means a light, vibrant day. You can eat as much fruit as you want during the morning, right up until about twenty to thirty minutes before you eat something else. Once you have eaten another food, three hours should elapse – at least – before anything else is eaten. Once again, listen to your body. When your stomach is empty, you can have more fruit.

Literally thousands of people from my seminars have stopped eating heavy foods in the morning and have just fruit and fruit juice. They have made incredible turnarounds. Many of them come to me and say, 'Listen, you know when I first heard this, I was a big breakfast eater, but I was willing to at least try what you said and then go back to eating breakfast.' They didn't, they couldn't go back to heavier breakfasts. If you want to know what it feels like to swallow an anvil, all you have to do is eat exclusively fruit and fruit juice in the morning for about ten days, and then try to go back to having a heavier meal in the morning. You simply won't do it. Yes, perhaps you will on occasion, and that is certainly okay. Because occasionally is one thing. Every day is something entirely different.

The consumption of exclusively fruit and fruit juice in the morning is at the very heart of **FIT FOR LIFE**.

Interestingly, many people have told me that although they don't adhere to the program exactly all the time, the one thing they do most consistently is adhere to the exclusive consumption of fruit and fruit juice before noon, because with that alone they still reap enormous benefits. It is without question the major contributing factor to the success of FIT FOR LIFE. If you are going to start with only one principle, this should be it. **FRUIT EXCLUSIVELY IN THE MORNING.**

Some people think that a lot of fruit and fruit juice is fattening. The only time fruit can cause any negative manifestations at all is when it is altered by heat or incorrectly combined, meaning consumed with or immediately following any other food. **WHEN EATEN ON AN EMPTY STOMACH, FRESH FRUIT CAN HAVE ONLY A POSITIVE EFFECT; IT ACCELERATES WEIGHT LOSS.** When we tell people they can freely eat more fruit than usual and make this a habit in their lives, some of them initially express concern over the amount of calories they are taking in. Calories are enemies only if they are consumed in foods that are highly processed or ill-combined. High-quality calories, those found in high-water-content food, are not going to add to your weight problem. They will furnish the energy to do away with it.

I have always found calorie-counting to be such a bore. It is a depressing way to determine what to eat. I implore people to forget about calories and think of high-quality food. Calorie-counting is a very antiquated and ineffective means of trying to regulate one's weight. It looks viable in theory, so does the theory that the sun orbits the earth. Calorie-counting is an unrealistic gauge by which to measure one's progress. That is why so many calorie-counters do not find the results they are looking for, even though they diligently count their calories.

I remember once going into a very nice restaurant in

Palm Springs for breakfast. This establishment prided itself on the fact that everything on the menu had the number of calories indicated next to it. Here is why calorie-counting is practically worthless: I worked out two possible breakfasts from the menu. Both had three items. One was 220 calories, the other 190. Well, if I were operating under the delusion that a calorie is a calorie is a calorie, and I should eat fewer at a meal whenever possible, I would have opted for the breakfast of 190 calories. But understanding the principles of Natural Hygiene as I did, I unhesitatingly had the 220-calorie breakfast. Lucky for me. You see, thinking that a calorie in a food that has been denatured, devitalized, and otherwise processed to death is just like a calorie in a fresh, unadulterated food is folly of the highest order. All cars are cars too. Would you rather have a broken-down old jalopy with no brakes that barely runs or a shiny new Rolls-Royce? Both are cars, but one can endanger your life while the other can serve it. So it is with calories. One kind can *add* weight to your body, another kind can supply the energy to help you *lose* weight. When dealing with calories, it is a classic instance of quality being of far greater importance than quantity.

The 190-calorie breakfast was a bowl of oatmeal, one piece of wheat toast, and cream cheese. The 220-calorie breakfast was a glass of fresh-squeezed orange juice, a slice of fresh melon in season, and a bowl of fresh strawberries. Now that you have a clear understanding of the extreme importance of eating foods high in water content, properly combined, I'm sure you can see why I opted for the 220-calorie meal. The 190-calorie breakfast was three items devoid of water. It was a protein (cream cheese) and two carbohydrates (toast and oatmeal). It would have sat rotting in my stomach for some six to eight hours, robbing me of my precious energy, supplying no nutrition, and leaving a thick layer of toxic waste to clog my system. It would have done absolutely nothing to assist in my desire to lose weight. It would have *added* weight. The 220-calorie breakfast was *all* high water content. No putrefaction or fermentation and the resulting distress to my system. It passed through my stomach in less than half an hour and was actually supplying me with real energy within an hour. My system was helped, not prevented from cleansing itself of waste, because my elimination cycle was not thwarted.

Anyone who would think that this program is successful because it supplies fewer calories than a 'regular' diet has missed the point of it entirely. Merely lowering calorie intake will not achieve the loss of weight desired if the calories consumed are from foods that are denatured, ill-combined, toxic, and clogging. That is why this program has been so successful for so many people, many of whom used to count calories religiously. It is a life-style change having nothing to do with calorie-counting.

The reasoning behind eating exclusively fruit in the morning is tied closely to the efficient functioning of your body cycles. This is a perfect time to look at these cycles again and see exactly why. Since in weight loss we are interested in not blocking the elimination cycle, let's emphasize that cycle by looking at it first.

CYCLE I – ELIMINATION (4 A.M.–NOON):
You have already learned that digestion of conventional food takes more energy than any other body process. You have also learned that fruit demands the least amount of energy for its digestion. So it is most beneficial for **FRUIT OR FRUIT JUICE TO BE THE ONLY FOODS CONSUMED DURING THE ELIMINATION CYCLE**, if you consume anything at all. Anything else halts the elimination

process, and the by-products of foods that should have been eliminated are now added to your toxic load and to the unwanted pounds in your body. That is why the success of this program (and your success in losing weight) depends on the exclusive consumption of fruit and fruit juice before noon. Successful and comfortable weight loss is dependent on the efficiency of the elimination cycle. By sabotaging this cycle you sabotage your success. **HAVING ONLY FRUIT AND FRUIT JUICE EXCLUSIVELY BEFORE NOON IS THE SINGLE MOST IMPORTANT FACET OF THIS SYSTEM.** (Even if you continue to drink coffee or take supplements, don't do it during the elimination cycle. Do it after noon. This is essential.)

CYCLE II - APPROPRIATION (NOON–8 P.M.):
After twelve o'clock we enter the daily eating period. If you are hungry, this is the time to eat, but there are some important rules to observe here. Remember that digestion takes more energy than anything else you do. You want to eat a meal that will not deplete your energy supply, even though it will demand *some* digestive energy. (See the Energy Ladder on page 198.) That means adhering to the principle of proper food combining so that a minimum of digestive energy is depleted to break down that meal.

CYCLE III - ASSIMILATION (8 P.M.–4 A.M.):
You have taken in the food. Now it is time to give your body a chance to extract, absorb, and utilize the nutrients in that food. No absorption can take place until the food has entered the intestines. A properly combined meal will be out of the stomach in approximately three hours and ready to be absorbed and assimilated. An improperly combined meal can remain in the stomach anywhere from eight to twelve hours or *longer*. Eat early enough so that food has left your stomach before

you retire. A full night's rest (beginning well before midnight as often as possible) will permit your body to complete the assimilation cycle before it again enters the elimination phase around 4 a.m.

Having been introduced to these tools and given the steps to bring about the success you are seeking, before going on it is imperative that you have a very clear understanding of . . .

CHAPTER 8

The Theory of Detoxification

We have been stressing throughout this book the extreme importance of eliminating toxic waste from the system to achieve successful, permanent weight loss. To facilitate that process we have developed a life-style that is not only effective, but also easy and comfortable.

The detoxification of your system is the most important goal of FIT FOR LIFE. Understand that the detoxification of your body is occasionally not the most pleasant phase of creating the environment for weight loss, although it is a necessary one. We don't want to lead you to believe that we have some miracle formula that will effortlessly transform you into a happy, healthy, slim individual overnight just by reading this book. You must do your part too. From experience over the last several years I can tell you that approximately 10 per cent of the people who make use of this information feel some degree of *initial* discomfort. There are certain *potential* discomforts, but they can definitely be minimized, If detoxification is too rapid, it can cause great discomfort. That is why over nine years have been spent experimenting and perfecting a life-style that can and does reduce this possible discomfort to the minimum.

It must be kept in mind that the building up of the toxic waste in your body may have taken twenty, thirty, forty, fifty years, or more, so its elimination is not something that is accomplished overnight. I cannot possibly overemphasize how exceedingly important it is for this detoxification to be accomplished. It is absolutely essential for the system to be cleansed so that energy can be freed up to be used in reducing weight. As long as there is toxic waste in the system, much of your available energy will be used to eliminate it. The success of any weight-loss program depends on the system being cleansed. Detoxification *is* cleansing and it *is* imperative! It's the key to the whole thing!

The possible discomforts depend on how toxic your system is. People who are particularly toxic or have taken drugs (prescription or not) on any regular basis are more apt to experience some temporary discomfort than those who are less toxic. The elimination of toxic waste *can* be uncomfortable. But better to have minor discomforts now than to have it all come crashing down on you, totally incapacitating you, at a later date. The important thing is for a person's diet to be such that cleansing takes place, but *not* at breakneck speed. It can be regulated so that the individual experiences the least amount of discomfort possible. This is precisely what the suggested menus later in the book succeed in doing. Be aware that these are *not just* menus. A tremendous amount of time, effort, study, and experimentation has gone into perfecting just the right blend of variables to assure that detoxification is as smooth and comfortable as possible. The FIT FOR LIFE program is, in fact, a detoxification program.

What are these possible discomforts? The most

frequent one is an initial bloating of the system. When you start to apply the principle of eating more fruit on an empty stomach, its cleansing ability will stir up accumulated toxic waste, creating gas and bloat. Generally this bloating passes within forty-eight hours. It rarely lasts longer than seventy-two hours. If this bloating should cause you to *add* two or three pounds during the first few days, it is *not* something to get alarmed about. The body is adjusting itself for the task ahead. You may experience headaches or body aches. You may feel suddenly tired or anxious. You may experience loose, runny stools that many people tend to equate with diarrhea. This is not something to become alarmed about or make you run out of the house for Kaopectate. Believe it or not, this loosening of the stools has a positive effect, not a negative one. The cleansing aspect of fruit washes impacted fecal matter from the intestinal walls and flushes it out of the system in the form of loose stools. This leaves you feeling light and renewed. It may be uncomfortable, but it serves a very beneficial purpose. It is imperative that you do not do anything to stop this (or any other) elimination process. Your body is ridding itself of toxic waste. Have no concerns about dehydrating. There is no temperature or signs of sickness involved with this elimination. With the amount of high-water-content fruits and vegetables you will be eating, there will be no possibility of that happening. To stop the elimination would mean keeping this waste in your system and insuring a weight problem. Loose stools rarely last more than two days. You may also experience some nausea as the toxins in your system are stirred up.

Perhaps you will have a copious discharge of mucus from your nasal passages. THIS IS NOT A 'COLD'! Your body is merely spewing out the excess toxins that have been built up and stored in the mucous membranes. One of the classic ways in which the human body eliminates toxicity is by means of what is called a cold. When the mucous membranes of your body become overladen with more mucus than the body can tolerate, and this mucus is not being eliminated as rapidly as it should, the defense mechanisms of the body take over to force it out through the throat and nose. If you took a glass and continuously poured water into it, it would eventually overflow. It is the same with your body. If there is more mucus in your body than it can accommodate, it will overflow.

Digestive disorders ranging from gas and flatulence to more serious chronic pains and colitis are a serious problem in this country. One of the major benefits from eating the way we teach in this book is that those problems will begin to be eradicated. Proper food combining and the correct consumption of fruit will be the major contributing factors to relieving these ills. On occasion the introduction of fruit, *properly eaten,* will cause some gas and flatulence. You may be eating fruit absolutely correctly (on an empty stomach in the morning) and still develop this gas and flatulence. The main reason this happens is that there is an accumulation of food debris and body wastes that have built up over the years and permeated the lining of the stomach and intestines. Fruit has the tendency to stir up and flush out this toxic matter. In the process, what is stirred up causes gas and flatulence. Most people never experience this situation, but I know a few who were particularly toxic and experienced it to a degree for two or three weeks. It all depends on how high or low the level of toxicity is in your body. In either case, even though it is uncomfortable and annoying, it is positive that the *cause* of the problem is being eliminated.

Keep in mind that any time you alter your eating

habits, your body has to adjust to that change and in so doing can initially leave you feeling out of sorts. The thing to do is **VIEW ANY TEMPORARY DISCOMFORT AS THE CLEANSING PROCESS TAKING PLACE AND HEALTH RETURNING.** You are witnessing health in action. The body is powerful and wants to 'get on with it' now that it has the chance. This can happen in many different forms. The body's reaction to having a sudden increase of energy at its disposal is to try to eliminate everything of a toxic nature as soon as possible while the energy is available. Once the system 'realizes' that this energy will be available on a regular basis, it starts to regulate the elimination, and the temporary discomfort disappears. **IT IS IMPORTANT TO REMEMBER THAT FEWER THAN 10 PER CENT OF THE PEOPLE WHO FOLLOW FIT FOR LIFE EXPERIENCE *ANY* DISCOMFORT.** Should you be one of those, *please* do not make the mistake of forsaking your new way of eating and returning to the old. This would throw your system into terrible turmoil. Have faith in the wisdom, intelligence, and wonderful recuperative abilities of your body, and be grateful that it has the integrity and capability to conduct a cleansing. Should any discomfort linger for more than a few days, to ease your mind and to be on the safe side, discuss it with your doctor or health adviser.

The total elimination of all toxicity from your body can take months or years, but within days you will be losing weight and feeling enormously more energetic and vibrant. The ongoing elimination usually continues without any outward manifestation or discomforts. Excess weight will be shed, energy will increase, everything will become progressively better. The biggest mistake you can make is to feel a little uncomfortable, say, 'The heck with it,' and return to your old eating habits. The discomfort you feel is an indication of how much you need to detoxify. It is a critical point and should not be thwarted. One thing is sure: Your body *wants* to cleanse out anything that is not helping to perpetuate your health. When it starts to come out, let it! You are far better off to have it outside your body than in your body. It is worth noting again that NOT EVERYONE FEELS DISCOMFORT. MOST PEOPLE HAVE NO PROBLEM WHATSOEVER. We just feel it is our responsibility to prepare you for the possibilities. If you are one of the many who don't experience discomfort, great! If not, the life-style presented on the following pages will keep discomfort at a minimum.

You can be absolutely certain that evidence supporting this plan of eating is abundant. For example, as mentioned earlier the number-one and number-two killer diseases in the United States are heart disease and cancer, respectively. Some four thousand people in the United States die *every day* from these two diseases! The very latest information coming from the scientific community is that an increase of fruits and vegetables in one's diet can decrease the incidence of both these killers. In September 1982 doctors at the National Cancer Institute said, 'Changing the way we eat could offer some protection against cancer. The first guideline is to reduce fat. The second is to increase the amount of fruits and vegetables. The National Cancer Institute has now made diet its number-one area of research in cancer prevention.' Also in September 1983 the American Cancer Society stated its belief that a 'greater use of fruits and vegetables can significantly reduce a person's risk of developing cancer.'

As indicated in the previous chapter, Dr Castelli of Harvard feels that heart disease risk could be cut by the consumption of fruit.

I am certain that fruits and vegetables can help lower the incidence of these problems, because these foods are so instrumental in detoxifying one's body. And the extent to which this detoxification assists in weight loss is tremendous.

By making use of these tools you are going to lose weight and keep that weight off. The only factors preventing you from making these simple changes are habits you may have. It's habit to eat a heavy meal in the morning. It's habit to mix proteins and carbohydrates. It's habit to eat fruit after meals. It is very important that we have some *new* habits. There's an old saying that if you don't get rid of some of your old habits, you're going to wind up where you're headed. And some of you don't *want* to wind up where you're headed now. The easiest way for you to get rid of old habits is to simply crowd them out with new and better ones.

This is exactly what we are providing here – a group of improved habits that you can use as much as you want or as little as you want. You don't have to do it so much that you feel as if you're under pressure. Take your time, enjoy yourself. This isn't something that you have to make into an ordeal. *And it is not a diet.* This is not a program to which you have to adhere to the letter. What we have provided you with is simply a way for you to respect the body's biological limitations and cycles. Considering what the experts are saying – that we need to eat more fruits and vegetables – we have provided you with a convenient way of doing just that. There is a fun way for you to experience the vibrant, good-looking body that you instinctively know should be yours.

This system is open for you to try at any pace you choose. It has been presented in such a way as to cause no problem if you make use of the information as little or as much as you desire. Some of you are going to be highly motivated, stick to the program exclusively, and experience the results you are looking for more rapidly than others. What we would like you to understand is that this is a lifelong program. This isn't two or four weeks' worth. This is information that is designed to stay with you, that you will incorporate into your life-style forever so you can start to experience the well-being that you deserve and that is your birthright.

You know life's gift to you is your body. Your thanks in return is to take the best care of it you can. Give it a chance to function at its highest level, unimpeded by toxic waste and weight. Your body wants to shine. It does not want to be overweight. It wants to have the shape that you know it can have. All you have to do is facilitate its natural processes, and you can start to experience the joys of a body you will be proud of. Enjoy yourself as you watch the emergence of the slender body you know has been locked inside you all this time.

I think you can see from what you have read in the principles so far that what is offered is not some hit-and-run scheme for quick, temporary results. These are principles to be incorporated into your life-style. Rather than a part-time diet scheme, you now have a full-time plan for life! You may be wondering, 'Can it be this simple? All I have to do is eat high-water-content foods, properly combine food, and eat fruit correctly? Will that do it?' YES! Yes, it will! The simply marvelous aspect of this is that it *is* just that simple. FIT FOR LIFE doesn't lock you into anything. You know the principles; you merely adhere to them as best you can. There's no 'blowing it.' You *can't* blow it. Just do the best you can when you can. As long as you do something good, you will reap the rewards. You have the rest of your life, so don't put undue pressure on yourself. If the principles make sense to you and you're willing to try them, that's all it will take. You have been given tools to use when you wish. You're in control. Like master woodcarvers who can go anywhere in the world and practice their trade, as long as they have their tools with them, **YOU CAN USE THE TOOLS OF FIT FOR LIFE WHEREVER YOU ARE, WHATEVER YOU ARE DOING, AND WHATEVER YOUR CIRCUMSTANCES.** The days of throwing your life into turmoil are over. No more locking up your refrigerator, taking diet pills, counting calories, or existing on measly portions. This is it! Liberation!

You can eat, and eat well, and you can enjoy your food. You can avoid putting yourself through another one of those self-depriving, self-defeating two- or four-week ordeals that bring you nothing but frustration and temporary results. You now have a realistic, lifelong approach that you can *live* with – literally!

Now that we have completed the principles, there are two areas of food consumption that demand attention because of their extreme influence on successful weight control and energy enhancement. The first of these is . . .

CHAPTER 9

Protein

Probably *the* most frequently asked question in the area of diet, health, and weight loss is 'Where do you get your protein?' The fear of dying in this country doesn't begin to compare with people's fear of not getting enough protein. The problem, however, is not how to get enough, it's how not to get too much. Having too much protein in one's body is easily as dangerous as not having enough.

In the words of Mike Benton of the American College of Health Science, 'Perhaps never have so many been so confused over a subject about which they know so little.'

I know what an exceedingly confusing topic this is. Everyone seems to have a different opinion as to how much protein should or should not be eaten and why. What always frustrated me was listening to a 'board-certified authority' discuss in a most convincing manner what I should know about protein. Then I would hear another equally authoritative 'expert' speak as convincingly as the first but say the exact *opposite*! That, I think, is the position most people are in. The experts are arguing up and back, burying the listener under an avalanche of facts, figures, statistics, and proof. The public winds up feeling like the ball in a tennis match. One thing in all of this is undeniably true: People are confused!

Right about now you may very well be asking, 'What makes you any different from all those who have added to the confusion?' Good question. It's certainly the one I would have asked. Perhaps nothing. But my intention is not to persuade you to accept what *I* know to be true, nor is it to totally reeducate you right here and now. To give you a clear understanding of the protein issue, it is going to take more than what I am about to relate. It is going to take some study and experimentation on your part. My intention is to get you to feel confident that *you* can make an intelligent decision for yourself, without having to depend on the experts who are arguing with one another. You already have the tools necessary to do so. And you know what those tools are: common sense, logic, and instinct. I will be appealing to your inherent ability to 'know' the right thing to do. You will have ample opportunity to exercise those tools by the end of this chapter.

There is a voluminous amount of information showing a relationship between the consumption of concentrated protein foods and heart disease, high blood pressure, cancer, arthritis, osteoporosis, gout, ulcers, and a host of other maladies, documented by T. C. Fry, Victoras Kulvinskas, Blanche Leonardo, Barbara Parham, John A. Scharffenberg, Orville Schell, and Herbert M. Shelton, among others. This discussion will, however, confine itself to the effects on one's weight and energy level.

Protein is the most complex of all food elements, and its assimilation and utilization are the most complicated. The easiest food for the body to break down is fruit; the other end of the scale, the hardest, is protein. When protein food is eaten, more energy is necessary for it to go through its process of digestion than for any other food. The average time for food (other than fruit) to pass through the entire gastrointestinal tract is between twenty-five and thirty hours. When flesh food is eaten, that time is *more* than doubled. Therefore, logically, the more protein one eats, the less energy will be available for other necessary functions, such as the elimination of toxic waste.

The entire protein issue has been blown so far out of proportion that it is doubtful that people will ever feel at ease with it. The bottom line is that we simply don't need as much as we have been led to believe.[1] First of all, the human body recycles 70 per cent of its proteinaceous waste. That's 70 per cent! Second, the human body loses only about twenty-three grams of protein a day. That's 8⁄10 of an ounce. It is lost through the feces, urine, hair, sloughed-off skin, and perspiration. To replenish 8⁄10 of an ounce you would need to eat about a pound and a half of protein a *month*. Most people eat far in excess of that, eating protein at every meal. The RDA protein requirement is 56 grams daily (less than two ounces!), and that is with their built-in safety margin of nearly doubling the actual need! Consuming more than the body requires places a heavy burden on the system as it tries to rid itself of this excess. It is a dreadful waste of your precious energy that is so dearly needed in the quest for weight loss. An 8-ounce glass can hold only 8 ounces of liquid. If you pour 16 ounces into the glass, everything over 8 ounces will go to waste. So it is with your body. Once the daily requirements are met, 8⁄10 of an ounce, that's it. Another

[1] Arthur C. Guyton. *Guidance Textbook of Medical Physiology.* Philadelphia: Saunders Publishing Co., 1981.

T. C. Fry. 'Lesson #8, Proteins in the Diet.' In *The Life Science Health System.* Austin, Texas: Life Science, 1983.

problem is that the excess protein not only robs you of your energy, but also must be stored in your body as toxic waste, adding weight until the organism can muster sufficient energy to get rid of it. But the next day there is another surplus to deal with, so the situation is worsened.

Actually protein is not any more or less important than any of the other constituents of food. We have been led to believe that one is more important, but that simply is not accurate. They all play a crucial role in making a food a food. Given a choice, which would you choose to give up if you had to choose one: your heart or your brain? It's the same with food. The constituents of foods that compose a typical meal are always the same. There are vitamins, minerals, carbohydrates, fatty acids, amino acids, and many more constituents that have yet to be isolated and named. They are *all* important! They are all used together synergistically. To single one out as more important than another is to fail to understand the biological and physiological needs of the organism.

No debate on protein would be complete without discussing meat-eating, because in this country meat is generally thought to be the most ideal source of protein. One of the major reasons is that animal protein much more closely resembles that of the human body than plant protein. It's an excellent argument for eating one's neighbor, actually, but even the heartiest meat-eater would find that idea repugnant.

One of the groups of animals that is eaten for protein is cattle, some thirty-three million a year. That's a lot of meat. For strength! That's usually the first reason given for the necessity of eating meat. 'We need to keep up our strength.' Well, let's just take a look at that. What would you say is the strongest animal on the planet? Most people would say an elephant. I would agree. As a matter of fact, if you had to think of the strongest animals in the world, the ones used for centuries for their superior strength and endurance, what would they be? Elephants, oxen, horses, mules, camels, water buffalo. What do they eat? Leafy matter, grass, and fruit. Have you ever seen a silverback gorilla? The silverback gorilla physiologically resembles the human being. It is incredibly strong. Even though one is 3 times the size of a man, it has 30 times a man's strength! A silverback could toss a 200-pound man across the street like a Frisbee. And what does the silverback eat? Fruits and other vegetation![2] What does that indicate to you about the necessity to eat meat for strength? Forget for the time being all the input and opinions you've heard. What do *you* think? What about the steer meat being eaten for its near-perfect protein? What did the steer eat to build that protein? Meat? No! Grain and grass! Interesting, isn't it? How can that be? On one side we have all the scientific data showing the benefits of eating meat, and on the other we have our common sense finding that point of view hard to swallow.

This brings us to the most misunderstood area of the entire question of meat-eating. The people who know the situation for what it is find this to be the most ironic aspect of this subject: Protein is not built in the body by eating protein. Yes, you read it correctly. Protein is built from the amino acids in food. The only extent to

[2] Two recognized authorities on the habits of gorillas are John Aspinal, who ran a world-famous refuge in England, and Adrien De Schryver. Both indicated that in their natural habitat gorillas are voracious fruit-eaters. In fact, when fruit is plentiful, they forgo the eating of any other food until the fruit is depleted. Mr. Aspinal was the subject of a program entitled 'Passion to Protect,' which P.B.S. aired on 19 August 1984. Mr. De Schryver was the subject of a program entitled 'The Man Who Lives with Gorillas,' aired by P.B.S. on 23 August 1984.

which protein is built from protein food is how well the amino acids in that food are utilized. The idea that you can eat a piece of steer or pig or chicken and that it will become protein in your body is absurd. Animal protein is just that: animal protein, not human protein. Amino acids must be understood if you wish to understand the protein issue.

The body cannot use or assimilate protein in its original state as eaten. The protein must first be digested and split into its component amino acids. The body can then use these amino acids to construct the protein it needs. The ultimate value of a food's protein, then, lies in its amino acid composition. It is the amino acids that are the essential components. All nutritive material is formed in the plant kingdom; animals have the power to appropriate but never to form or create protein's source, the eight essential amino acids. Plants can synthesize amino acids from air, earth, and water, but animals, including humans, are dependent on plant protein – either directly, by eating the plant, or indirectly, by eating an animal that has eaten the plant. There are no 'essential' amino acids in flesh that the animal did not derive from plants, and that humans cannot also derive from plants. That is why all the animals of strength have all the protein they need. They build it from the abundance of amino acids that they consume eating plant life. This is also why, except in emergencies, carnivorous animals generally don't eat other carnivorous animals. They instinctively eat animals that have eaten plant life.

There are 23 different amino acids. *All* are essential, or they wouldn't exist. As it happens, 15 can be produced by the body and 8 must be derived from the foods we eat. Only these 8 are called *essential*. If you eat any fruits, vegetables, nuts, seeds, or sprouts on a regular basis, you are receiving all the amino acids necessary for your body to build the protein it needs, just like the other mammals who seem to manage without eating meat. The fact is you couldn't have a protein deficiency unless you worked hard at having one. Do you know anyone with a protein deficiency? I don't either.

Now, don't let the amino acid issue confuse you. All that talk about having to eat all the essential amino acids at one meal or at least in one day is pure balderdash. There is no question but that this is the most controversial subject in this book. I know that the belief that the need for the 'eight essentials' at every meal has been nutritional gospel for years, but there is strong evidence mounting that this is not the case. Well-meaning books like *Diet for a Small Planet,* while convincing people to consume less meat, have succeeded in raising undue anxieties about satisfying the body's amino acid requirements. I personally have had to allay the fears of hundreds of people who have come to me wondering about protein deficiencies now that they have cut back on their meat and dairy intake. Trying to apply the complicated formulas in that book, they were finding themselves confused about their protein intake. I have also personally verified through the numbers of people I have counseled that the theories requiring all the amino acids at every meal result in unnecessary weight problems. People end up eating far too much concentrated food! (NOTE: In the words of Frances Moore Lappé, the author of *Diet for a Small Planet,* 'I went overboard on the precision angle. I was trying to please all the doctors and nutritionists, to be sure the book was beyond scientific reproach. I think I made people too self-conscious about combining proteins . . . be relaxed with it, most of us don't have to worry about protein anyway.')[3]

Common sense makes me ask why humans would be the only animal species to have such a complicated time of it obtaining the necessary components of protein. No animal in nature needs to combine different foods to get all the essentials. It is my contention that the reason it is so complicated for humans is because humans are the only animals with the ability to reason, and we have made it far more complicated for ourselves than it actually is.

Merely because something has been believed for a very long time does not make it true. For example, in 1914 Robert Bárány won a Nobel prize in physiology and medicine for his theory that relates to the workings of the inner ear and the body's balance mechanisms. In December 1983 a test aboard the Space Shuttle showed his theory to be false. Even though it was being taught in colleges throughout the world, in one fell swoop it was disproven. The fact that it was taught for nearly three quarters of a century did not make it true. Now the textbooks must be revised. I have powerful sources to back me up on the issue of protein, but remember, it took only *one* test to destroy a 70-year-old belief that a simple inner ear test could evaluate a person's equilibrium – a test routinely used by otolaryngologists (ear, nose, and throat specialists) for decades. The information stated here will make obsolete the present theories governing amino acids and how we get them. Time will prove this to be true.[4]

[3] Quoted in *The Vegetarian Child* by Joy Gross. Secaucus, New Jersey: Lyle Stuart, Inc., 1983: 55–56.

[4] Arthur C. Guyton. *Physiology of the Body*. Philadelphia: W. B. Saunders, 1964. T. C. Fry. *The Life Science Health System*. Austin, Texas: College of Life Science, 1983. Victoras Kulvinskas. *Survival into the 21st Century*. Wethersfield, Connecticut: Omangod Press, 1975.

You will recall the discussion earlier of the infinite wisdom of your body. It knows full well how to insure itself adequate protein production. How could it be otherwise? The body has a most remarkable mechanism to guarantee that something as crucial as protein is manufactured regularly and with great proficiency. That is the amino acid pool.

From the digestion of foods in the diet and from the recycling of proteinaceous wastes, the body has all the different amino acids circulating in the blood and lymph systems. When the body needs amino acids, they are appropriated from the blood or lymph. This continuous circulating available supply of amino acids is known as the amino acid pool. The amino acid pool is like a bank that is open 24 hours. The liver and cells are continually making deposits and withdrawals of amino acids, depending upon the concentration of amino acids in the blood.

When the number of amino acids is high, the liver absorbs and stores them until needed. As the amino acid level in the blood falls due to withdrawals by the cells, the liver deposits some of the stored amino acids back into circulation.

The cells also have the capacity to store amino acids. If the amino acid content of the blood falls, or if some other cells require specific amino acids, the cells are able to release their stored amino acids into circulation. Since most of the body's cells synthesize more protein than is necessary to support the life of the cell, the cells can reconvert their proteins into amino acids and make deposits into the amino acid pool. This pool of amino acids is critical to understanding why complete proteins are not necessary in the diet.

I know it sounds a bit involved, but relax, that's about as technical as I will ever get in this book. The amino acid pool exists, and understanding it will free you from the onerous protein myth.

The existence of the amino acid pool is by no means a new discovery. Much of the information about diet today is based on outmoded data that has not been updated. New knowledge has completely reversed the old theory, which was based on studies between 1929 and 1950 that used purified amino acids. We eat foods – not purified amino acids. My studies and many others since 1950[5] have shown that it is not necessary to eat complete proteins at every meal or even every day. A study conducted by E. S. Nasset, detailed in *World Review of Nutrition and Dietetics,* reported that 'the body can make up any of the amino acids missing in a particular meal from its own pool of reserves, as long as a variety of foods are included in the diet.'

Presenting strong evidence for the amino-acid-pool theory are the books on physiology by Arthur C. Guyton. His books are the standard physiological texts in colleges in this country. As early as 1964, in his *Physiology of the Body,* he discussed the amino acid pool and the body's ability to recycle proteinaceous waste.

T. C. Fry, the dean of the American College of Health Science, is another authority on this matter. His Life Science Health System course teaches the amino-acid-pool theory. This information has been available for over twenty years and is now coming to light. The main reason this information is being questioned is because it does not fit into the mold of what has traditionally

[5] C. Paul Bianchi and Russell Hilf. *Protein Metabolism and Biological Function.* New Brunswick, New Jersey: Rutgers University Press, 1970.

Henry Brown, M.D. *Protein Nutrition.* Springfield, Illinois: Charles C. Thomas Publishers, 1974.

H. N. Munro et al. *Mammalian Protein Metabolism.* New York: Academic Press, 1970: 4.

been taught. It seems that new information is usually rejected before it is accepted. There will always be new information filtering down from the enormous body of knowledge that I refer to as the great unknown. To scrutinize it is fine. To condemn it without investigation is folly. In addition to scientific verification, this information can be verified simply by putting it into practice. People who eat this way over long periods of time or even *lifetimes* have NO protein problems. The Hunzas, Vilcabambans, Asians, and half a billion Hindus eat very little protein food in comparison with Western populations, yet have no protein deficiencies. And not surprisingly, no weight problems!

There are 8 amino acids that the body must appropriate from outside sources, and although all fruit and vegetables contain most of the eight, there are many fruits and vegetables that contain *all* the amino acids not produced by the body: carrots, bananas, brussels sprouts, cabbage, cauliflower, corn, cucumbers, eggplant, kale, okra, peas, potatoes, summer squash, sweet potatoes, and tomatoes. Also all nuts, sunflower and sesame seeds, peanuts, and beans contain all eight as well.

You might be interested to know that the utilizable amino acid content found in plant life is far in excess of that to be found in flesh foods. I know it must sound like I'm going to try to make a vegetarian of everyone. Actually that's not my intent, although, in the words of Albert Einstein, 'It is my view that the vegetarian manner of living, by its purely physical effect on the human temperament, would most beneficially influence the lot of mankind.' As you've probably guessed, I'm a vegetarian. I learned a long time ago that it's a lot easier to sneak up on plants. But I do not want to force vegetarianism on anyone not interested in it. You can still eat some meat and maintain health. I know some vegetarians who think just because they don't eat meat, they have carte blanche to eat anything else they desire. They subsequently are far unhealthier than some rational meat-eaters I know.

The question should be: Are human beings designed and intended to eat meat? What all the available evidence points to is that there is no nutritional, physiological, or psychological justification for meat-eating by humans. Whoa! Okay, pick yourself up off the floor and I'll explain.

First let's look at the nutritional aspects of flesh food. As indicated earlier, the number-one prerequisite of a food is most certainly its fuel value, fuel as it relates to energy for the body's use. Flesh foods supply *no* fuel, *no* energy. Fuel is built from carbohydrates. Meat has virtually *no* carbohydrates. In other words, **NO FUEL VALUE**. Fats may supply energy, but they must undergo a longer and less efficient digestive process, and fats may be converted into fuel only when **THE BODY'S CARBOHYDRATE RESERVES ARE DEPLETED**. It should be understood that fat in the body does not all come from the fat that is eaten in the diet. When an excess of carbohydrates is eaten, it is converted by the body into fat and stored. In this way the body can store and use fat without having a large amount of fat in the diet. The fat deposits could be viewed as a type of carbohydrate bank, where deposits and withdrawals are made as necessary. So *utilizable* fat is ultimately dependent upon carbohydrate intake.

Another consideration is fiber. Every area of health care is stressing the importance of fiber in the diet. Among other things, fiber helps to avoid constipation and hemorrhoids. Meat has virtually no fiber content.

Now let's look at the availability of amino acids in flesh food. An amino acid chain can contain anywhere from fifty-one to two hundred thousand amino acids.

When flesh protein is ingested, the chain has to be broken down and reassembled into *human* protein. Amino acids are somewhat delicate. The heat of cooking coagulates or destroys many of the amino acids so that they are not available for body use.[6] These unusable amino acids become toxic, adding to one's weight, increasing the chores of the body, and depleting energy. Meat would have to be eaten raw, the way carnivorous and omnivorous animals eat it, for any potential usage of amino acids. Except for the latest sushi rage, which has it own drawbacks,[7] people are not exactly eating their meat raw. Meat is also very high in saturated fat. Not the kind to be used for energy – the kind that causes heart attacks! So nutritionally, notwithstanding all the propaganda to the contrary, meat has very little, if anything, going for it.

Now let's look at the physiological aspects of meat-eating. A carnivore's teeth are long, sharp, and pointed – all of them! We have molars for crushing and grinding. A carnivore's jaw moves up and down *only,* for tearing and biting. Ours move from side to side for grinding. A carnivore's saliva is acid and geared to the digestion of animal protein; it lacks ptyalin, a chemical that digests starches. Our saliva is alkaline and contains ptyalin for

[6] A. Okitani et al. 'Heat Induced Changes in Free Amino Acids on Manufactured Heated Pulps and Pastes from Tomatoes.' *The Journal of Food Science* 48 (1983): 1366–1367.

E. J. Bigwood. *Protein and Amino Acid Functions.* New York: Pergamon Press, 1972.

C. E. Bodwell, Ph.D. *Evaluation of Proteins for Humans.* Westport, Connecticut: The Air Publishing Co., 1977.

T. C. Fry. 'Lesson #8, Proteins in the Diet.' In *The Life Science Health System.* Austin, Texas: Life Science, 1983.

[7] Sushi is always ill-combined – meat and rice, a protein and a starch – and raw fish is often blamed for the rise of intestinal worms in humans. In addition, raw fish is a storehouse for industrial pollutants from the water.

the digestion of starch. A carnivore's stomach is a simple round sack that secretes 10 times more hydrochloric acid than that of a noncarnivore. Our stomachs are oblong in shape, complicated in structure, and convoluted with a duodenum. A carnivore's intestines are 3 times the length of its trunk, designed for rapid expulsion of foodstuff, which quickly rots. Our intestines are 12 times the length of our trunks and designed to keep food in them until all nutrients are extracted. The liver of a carnivore is capable of eliminating 10 to 15 times more uric acid than the liver of a noncarnivore. Our livers have the capacity to eliminate only a small amount of uric acid. Uric acid is an extremely dangerous toxic substance that can wreak havoc in your body. All meat consumption releases large quantities of uric acid into the system. Unlike carnivores and most omnivores, humans do *not* have the enzyme uricase to break down uric acid. A carnivore does not sweat through the skin and has no pores. We do sweat through the skin and have pores. A carnivore's urine is acid. Ours is alkaline. A carnivore's tongue is rough. Ours is smooth. Our hands are perfectly designed for plucking fruit from a tree, not for tearing the guts out of the carcass of a dead animal as are a carnivore's claws.

There is not one anatomical faculty the human being has that would indicate that it is equipped for tearing, ripping, and rending flesh for consumption.

Lastly, we as humans are not even psychologically equipped to eat meat. Have you ever strolled through a lush wooded area, filling your lungs with good air while listening to the birds sing? Perhaps it was after a rain, and everything was fresh and clean. The sun was filtering through the trees and glistening off the moisture on the flowers and grass. Just then perhaps a chipmunk scurried across your path. What was your **VERY FIRST INSTINCTIVE** inclination upon the sight of the chipmunk, before you even had time to think? To pounce on it, grab it with your teeth, rip it apart, and swallow it, blood, guts, skin, bone, flesh, and all? Then lick your lips with delight and thank the powers that be that you chose this particular path through the woods so you had the opportunity to devour this delectable little tidbit? *Or* would you instantly, upon sight of the furry little creature, say, 'Shhh, did you see that cute little chipmunk?' I wonder how many more vegetarians there would be if when people wanted a piece of steak, they had to go out, beat a defenseless steer to death, cut it open, and wade through the blood and guts to slice out the particular parts they desired.

Kids are the real test. Place a small child in a crib with a rabbit and an apple. If the child eats the rabbit and plays with the apple, I'll buy you a new car.

So, why *do* people eat flesh? Two very simple reasons: number one, habit and conditioning – if hundreds of billions of dollars were spent regularly to convince people that if they cut off their feet they would never stub their toes, probably some would see the virtue of that way of thinking; number two, some people happen to like meat. And that's it. Which is all right as long as people aren't convinced that they eat meat for health reasons, because the only effect meat-eating has on health is that it deteriorates it. It demands a tremendous amount of energy to digest it, and it makes the task of losing weight more of a chore than it should be.

If you *do* wish to continue eating meat, I would like to offer three simple hints on how to minimize its negative effects:

1) Seek a good source. Some of the chemicals given to animals destined for slaughter are dangerous. These can include penicillin, tetracycline, sewage-sludge pellets decontaminated with cesium-137, radioactive nuclear waste, fattening agents, a host of other chemicals and antibiotics to 'prime' the animal for sale. Not to mention the chemical treatment some meat receives when it is routinely dipped in sodium sulphite to decrease the stench of decay and turn it red rather than the gray of dead flesh. Even cement dust! That's right! *Nutrition Health* reported in 1981 that some cattle farmers in the Midwest were feeding their steers hundreds of pounds of cement dust to get their weight up for sale. A consumer group, hearing of this ploy, complained to the FDA to halt it, and the FDA's statement after investigation was that since there has been no indication of harm to humans by ingesting some cement dust, the practice can continue until some harm is proved. Can you imagine trying to lose weight while you're eating cement dust? I don't like it. There are places that guarantee that their beef and chicken are naturally grazed and raised with absolutely *no* chemical additives at all. Seek out these sources. You're worth it. If your butcher doesn't carry it, ask for it.

2) Try to eat flesh no more than once a day. If meat is eaten more than once a day, the enormous amount of energy necessary to digest it would not leave sufficient energy for other important body functions, such as elimination. The one meat meal should be late in the day in accordance with the Energy Ladder on page 198. And some days don't have any flesh food at all. Don't worry, you'll wake up the next day. Probably with more spunk than the day before.

3) **PROPERLY COMBINE.** There are times when you will eat foods that are not properly combined. But try not to let it be a time when you are having flesh food. Flesh food combined properly places enough of a burden on the body; don't complicate it.

Some of you who are athletes might be saying, 'But I need more protein, because I'm active.' The following interesting comment appeared in a 1978 issue of the *Journal of the American Medical Association.* The Association's Department of Foods and Nutrition commented: 'The ingestion of protein supplements by athletes who eat an otherwise well-balanced diet is of no use in body-building programs. Athletes need the same amount of protein foods as nonathletes. Protein does not increase strength. Indeed, it often takes greater energy to digest and metabolize the excess of protein. In addition, excess protein in the athlete can induce dehydration, loss of appetite, and diarrhea.'[8]

If more physical activity is anticipated, it is necessary only to increase your carbohydrate intake to insure more fuel. Proteins are disastrous in fuel efficiency and do not aid directly or efficiently in muscular activity. Protein does not produce energy, *it uses it!* A lion, which eats exclusively flesh, sleeps twenty hours a day. An orangutan, which eats exclusively plants, sleeps six. Also, the *Journal of the American Medical Association* reported in 1961, 'A vegetarian diet can prevent 90 to 97 per cent of heart disease.'[9] That's quite a statistic.

One last issue must be addressed: vitamin B_{12}. Supposedly, if you don't eat meat, you'll develop a vitamin B_{12} deficiency. Poppycock! Where do the animals whose meat we eat get theirs? Vitamin B_{12} is found in plants in very small amounts. But the way vitamin B_{12} is secured is primarily *from that produced*

[8] Cyborski, Cathy Kapica. 'Protein Supplements and Body Building Programs.' *Journal of the American Medical Association* 240 (1978): 481.

[9] 'Diet and Stress in Vascular Disease.' *Journal of the American Medical Association* 176 (1961): 134.

in the body. The stomach secretes a substance called 'intrinsic factor,' which transports the vitamin B_{12} created by the bacterial flora in our intestines. The vitamin B_{12} issue is part and parcel of the entire protein myth. **WHERE DO THE CATTLE THAT SUPPLY US THE MEAT AND MILK GET THEIR B_{12}?** Supposedly we will perish without meat or dairy products. Without any sources to show this false except our common sense, we could discount it. However, there are numerous sources, some of which are listed below.[10] Our actual need for vitamin B_{12} is so minute that it is measured in micrograms (millionth of a gram) or nanograms (billionth of a gram). One milligram of vitamin B_{12} will last you over two years, and healthy individuals usually carry around a 5-year supply. But here's the rub: Putrefaction hampers the secretion of 'intrinsic factor' in the stomach and retards the production of vitamin B_{12}. So flesh-eaters are more apt to develop a vitamin B_{12} deficiency than vegetarians! This has been known for some time and was discussed in part in a report entitled 'Vitamins of the B Complex,' in the *1959 United States Department of Agriculture Year-book.* The propaganda states just the opposite!

You may be wondering if eggs fare any better than

[10] T. C. Fry. 'Lesson #32, Why We Should Not Eat Meat.' In *The Life Science Health System.* Austin, Texas: Life Science, 1984.

Paavo Airola. 'Meat for B_{12}?' *Nutrition Health Review.* Summer 1983: 13.

Robin A. Hur. *Food Reform – Our Desperate Need.* Herr-Heidelberg, 1975.

Viktoras Kulvinskas. *Survival into the 21st Century.* Wethersfield, Connecticut: Omangod Press, 1975.

R. P. Spencer. *The Intestinal Tract.* Springfield, Illinois: Charles Thomas, Publ., 1960.

D. K. Benerjee and J. B. Chatterjea. 'Vitamin B_{12} Content of Some Articles of Indian Diet and Effect of Cooking on It.' *British Journal of Nutrition* 94 (1968): 289.

flesh foods as a source for protein. Actually high-quality protein is not what we should search for. High-quality amino acids are what we need to *produce* the protein we must have. Unless eggs are eaten raw, the amino acids are coagulated by heat and thereby lost. Even if they are eaten raw, eggs are laid by hens that are fed arsenic to kill parasites and stimulate egg production, and you ingest some of that virulent poison. Also eggs contain much sulfur, which puts a heavy strain on the liver and kidneys. The beautiful human body does not require anything that stinks for its survival. Eggs stink. Just drop one on your driveway on a hot day and let it sit there for about eight hours, then take a big whiff of the effluvium. There's no difference between that and putting eggs in your body at 98.6 degrees for 8 hours. The next bowel movement after the consumption of eggs will certainly bear this out. Excuse me for being rude, but the facts must be acknowledged.

The tremendous need for protein was dealt a heavy blow by the International Society for Research on Nutrition and Vital Statistics, which is composed of 400 doctors of medicine, biochemistry, nutrition, and natural science. At a 1980 seminar in Los Angeles I came into contact with its report that our classical protein requirement tables need an overhaul. Meat, fish, and eggs supplement a basic diet, but a daily intake of these foods is not necessary.[11] Do you know how convincing the evidence had to be for this particular group to make this statement?

Dr Carl Lumholtz, a Norwegian scientist, conducted extensive studies of anthropophagy (cannibalism). He indicated that some aborigine tribes in Australia would

[11] This organization is now called The International Society for Research on Civilization and Environment. The address is 61 Rue E. Bouillot, BTE 11, B-1060 Brussels, Belgium.

not eat the flesh of Caucasians because it was salty and occasioned nausea. But Asians and other native tribesmen were considered good eating because their food was chiefly vegetable.[12]

To maintain your life and add life to your life, it is best to predominate your diet with those foods that are *full of life*! Incidentally, the word *vegetable* comes from the word *vegetus,* which means **FULL OF LIFE**!

Now that the subject of protein has been explained in its relationship to weight loss and energy, the other equally important factor in this area is . . .

[12] George M. Gould, M.D. and Walter L. Pyle, M.D. *Anomalies and Curiosities of Medicine*. New York: The Julian Press, 1956: 407. Original copyright 1896.

CHAPTER 10

Dairy Products

The advisability of eating dairy products is every bit as controversial as the habit of meat-eating. It is my opinion, after fifteen years of study, that aside from flesh food nothing will sabotage a successful, *healthy* weight-loss plan more quickly than eating dairy products. Here again I am trying to smash another belief system to smithereens. I know how hard it will be for some people to agree with me. I can just hear someone saying, 'Hey, if that includes Häagen-Dazs, forget it, pal!' Perhaps in the past you went on a regimen of *nothing but* meat and dairy and lost weight. I did too! I remember once eating absolutely nothing but eggs, meat, and cheese for one month! I lost 25 pounds. But I'll tell you what: I felt lousy, and one month after I returned to a 'regular' diet I had put the 25 pounds right back on. I was able to lose the weight because anytime a complete food group or two is removed from the diet, the body will lose weight. Simply by having less to deal with, my system lost weight. But because the things I was eating were devoid of water content, I didn't feel good, I was bored beyond belief, and my breath smelled like an accident at a sewage plant. Surely I wouldn't entertain the idea of eating nothing but eggs, meat, and cheese for the rest of my life.

More dairy products are consumed in the United States than in any other country in the world! In a survey by *Grocers Journal of California* in September 1982 it was reported that 'Dairy products have the highest incidence of consumption of any major food category. Only 6 per cent of Americans say they don't consume milk in some form.'

If dairy products are such good foods, and we in America eat more than any other country in the world, then it stands to reason that we should be experiencing the highest level of health as well. As a matter of fact, the American worker leads the world in degenerative diseases, according to Richard O. Keeler, Director of Program Development for the President's Council on Physical Fitness, reported in the *Los Angeles Times* in April 1981.

As with protein, there is a colossal amount of information linking the consumption of dairy products to heart disease, cancer, arthritis, migraine headaches, allergies, ear infections, colds, hay fever, asthma, respiratory ailments, and a multitude of other problems, as documented by Hannah Allen, Alec Burton, Viktoras Kulvinskas, F. M. Pottenger, Herbert M. Shelton, and N. W. Walker, among others. For our purposes here, dairy products are discussed only to the extent that they affect weight loss and energy.

You can be absolutely certain of one thing: Milk is the most political food in America. According to the *Los Angeles Times,* the dairy industry is subsidized (meaning the taxpayers foot the bill) to the tune of almost three billion dollars a year! That's 342,000 dollars *every hour* to buy hundreds of millions of dollars' worth of dairy products that will in all likelihood never be eaten. They are sitting in storage, and some of them are rotten to the core. The storage bill alone for the surplus that will never be used is 47 million dollars annually! The demand for dairy products has declined substantially, as it is becoming more apparent that they are not the perfect foods they were once touted to be.

But production is continuous. Be assured that much of the publicity referring to the health benefits of dairy products is commercially motivated. In March 1984 the *Los Angeles Times* reported that the Department of Agriculture decided to launch a $140-million advertising campaign 'to promote milk-drinking and help reduce the multibillion-dollar surplus.' Although the *real* reason for the advertising campaign is to reduce the surplus, the ads attempt to convince you to buy milk for its many so-called health benefits.

Arguing the pros and cons of eating dairy products would prove futile, so once again you will have to rely heavily on your own common sense in making a decision.

Let's get right to it. I will ask you a question that I wish for you to answer strictly from common sense. Cows don't drink cow's milk, so why do humans? What in the world are humans doing drinking cow's milk? If a grown cow was offered milk, it would sniff it and say, 'No, thanks, I'll have the grass.' Think about it. Could our creator possibly have set things up in such a way that the *only* species on earth to drink cow's milk would be human beings? Perhaps you are thinking to yourself, 'What's he talking about, calves drink cow's milk!' *Exactly!* Cow's milk was designed and created for one purpose and one purpose only: *to feed the young of the species.* No animals drink or want to drink milk once they are weaned. Of course, I am not talking about domesticated animals, who have been perverted from their natural inclinations. During the initial phase of life it is the invariable practice of *all mammals* to take the milk of their mothers; then they are weaned and spend the remainder of their lives sustained by other foods. Nature dictates that we are to be weaned at an early age. Humans, on the other hand, teach that after a mother has performed her nursing, the cow should take over. In other words, there is *one* mammal on earth that should never, ever be weaned: humans! *Why?* Of course, it is difficult to look at the issue objectively, because of all the contradictory information that abounds, but isn't your sense of logic and your common sense a bit offended by the idea that humans should never be weaned?

Have you ever seen a zebra nursing off a giraffe? No? Have you ever seen a dog nursing off a horse? No? Well, have you ever seen a human nursing off a cow? All three examples are equally ridiculous. But you have seen humans nursing off cows, because if you have ever seen anyone drinking milk or eating any other kind of dairy product, you *have* seen it. Just because someone milks the cow and gets it to the consumer in a clean glass doesn't mean that person is not nursing from a cow. Of course, it doesn't seem strange at all to see someone drinking a glass of milk, but what would your reaction be if you were driving down some country lane and you happened to look over into one of the pastures to see a well-dressed man or woman down on his or her knees, suckling from a cow? Would *you* make your way through the droppings and go right up to a cow and take the milk directly from her udder? No? But you will let someone else get it and bring it to you in a glass, right? Of course, I'm being facetious, but it seems funny only because people's logic, instincts, and common sense would stop them from drinking milk if it were not supplied for them.

The facts are clear about one thing: The chemical composition of cow's milk is different from that of human's milk. If your insides could talk after you ingested a dairy product, they would ask, 'What's this person doing, hanging around cows?'

The enzymes necessary to break down and digest milk are renin and lactase. They are all but gone by the age of three in most humans. There is an element in all milk known as casein. There is 300 times more casein in cow's milk than in human's milk. That's for the development of huge bones. Casein coagulates in the stomach and forms large, tough, dense, difficult-to-digest curds that are adapted to the four-stomach digestive apparatus of a cow. Once inside the human system, this thick mass of goo puts a tremendous burden on the body to somehow get rid of it. In other words, a huge amount of energy must be spent in dealing with it. Unfortunately some of this gooey substance hardens and adheres to the lining of the intestines and prevents the absorption of nutrients into the body. Result: lethargy. Also the by-products of milk digestion leave a great deal of toxic mucus in the body. It's very acidic, and some of it is stored in the body until it can be dealt with at a later time. The next time you are going to dust your home, smear some paste all over everything and see how easy it is to dust. Dairy products do the same to the inside of your body. That translates into more weight instead of weight loss. Casein, by the way, is the base of one of the strongest glues used in woodworking.

Dr Norman W. Walker, the 109-year-old health specialist referred to earlier, has studied this subject for well over half a century and considers himself an expert on the glandular system. He states that a major contributing factor to thyroid problems is casein. The fact that dairy products are highly processed and always have traces of penicillin and antibiotics in them places even more of a burden on your system.

Many people are allergic to antibiotics, and no one suggests taking drugs *when well.* One should endeavor to ingest as few drugs as possible. The body must expend energy to break them down and remove them. In the *New England Journal of Medicine,* Doctors Holmberg, Osterholm, et al., reported that 'The widespread practice of feeding antibiotics to cattle to speed their growth creates potentially deadly bacteria that can infect humans. Seventeen persons became sick and one died because a herd of South Dakota cattle was fed antibiotics.'[1] In an editorial in the same issue Dr Stuart Levy, the senior editor of the journal, said, 'Surely the time has come to stop gambling with antibiotics. Although their use as feed additives had a major role in advancing livestock production in the past, the consequences of this practice are now too evident to overlook.'[2] It was pointed out that 'thousands of pounds of antibiotics were used in the fifties. Today it is millions of pounds.' The danger is there!

The most serious difficulty with dairy consumption is the formation of mucus in the system. It coats the mucous membranes and forces everything to transpire in a very sluggish fashion. Vital energy is always being squandered. It is a situation that must be rectified and avoided. Weight loss is made two or three times more difficult when the system is overladen with mucus.

Have you ever talked to people who every ten words or so make a kind of guttural sound as they try to release the mucus from behind their noses? Sounds something

[1] Holmberg, Osterholm, et al. 'Drug Resistant Salmonella from Animals Fed Antimicrobials.' *New England Journal of Medicine* 311 (1984): 617.
[2] Stuart Levy. 'Playing Antibiotic Pool.' *New England Journal of Medicine* 311 (1984): 663.

like *slurf!* The next time you meet a person like that, inquire as to what extent he or she eats dairy products. The chances of the answer being seldom or never is very small!

One of the most outspoken authorities challenging the traditional view of dairy products is Dr William A. Ellis, a retired osteopathic physician and surgeon. Dr Ellis is a highly respected individual in the scientific community and has researched milk and its related problems for 42 years! The link he shows between dairy products and heart disease, arthritis, allergies, and migraine headaches is impressive. He also makes two other important points. First, he says that there is 'overwhelming evidence that milk and milk products are a major factor in obesity.' Second, he states, 'Over my forty-two years of practice, I've performed more than twenty-five thousand blood tests for my patients. These tests show, conclusively, in my opinion, that adults who use milk products do not absorb nutrients as well as adults who don't. Of course, poor absorption, in turn, means chronic fatigue.'[3]

Now, all these problems exist even if dairy products are eaten properly combined. Since any dairy product is a concentrated food, no other concentrated food should be eaten with it. However, milk is usually consumed with a meal or with cake or cookies, or in oatmeal – all violations of proper food combining. Cheese is usually eaten on crackers, or in a sandwich, or with fruit – all violations of proper food combining. Taken alone, dairy products are enough of a hindrance to the body, but improperly combined they are a catastrophe. And, yes, this includes yogurt. *What?* 'Why, yogurt is a health food!' Hardly. It is made from cow's

[3] Samuel Biser. 'The Truth About Milk.' *The Healthview Newsletter,* 14. Charlottesville, Virginia (Spring 1978): 1-5.

milk, and cow's milk is for baby cows. The friendly bacteria you are supposedly getting when you eat yogurt are something that your body already produces in quantities about which it knows best. All that business about Russians living to be 130 years old by eating one of the current commercial yogurts is a joke. They never saw that product before the film crew showed up with their cameras. It's plenty of fresh air, hard physical labor, pure water, and pure foods raised by their own hands that contribute to their longevity![4]

If you are going to eat dairy products, please combine them properly for the least amount of detriment. Milk should be taken absolutely alone. It's *the* most mucous-forming food on the planet, and it doesn't go well with anything. If you want cheese, either chop it up in chunks and have it in a salad (without croutons) or melt some over some vegetables. Don't eat yellow cheeses, because they're soaked in chemical dyes. There may be some pizza fans out there who are getting ready to tear out these pages. If you want pizza once in a while, fine. At least be aware of the potential harm it causes and don't abuse it. If you have pizza one day, the next day clean up. Do what is in the best interest of your organism. Want some Häagen-Dazs? Don't have it right after a spicy Italian meal. Have it once in a while on an empty stomach so your system will at least have a fighting chance.

Same with yogurt. Don't have it with fruit on the bottom; it will all ferment and putrefy in your system. Have it plain on an empty stomach, or make it into a salad dressing. Fix a salad and mix yogurt through it.

Some people insist that dairy products are necessary for calcium. We're led to believe that milk is a major

[4] The Russians do eat yogurt, but in small amounts. The yogurt is quite fresh, and it is not fermented to the degree that commercial yogurt is.

source of calcium, and if we don't drink milk, our teeth will fall out and our bones will collapse. First of all, the calcium in cow's milk is much coarser than in human's milk, and is tied up with the casein. This prevents the calcium from being absorbable. Second, most milk-drinkers and cheese-eaters consume pasteurized, homogenized, or otherwise processed products. This processing degrades the calcium, making it very difficult to utilize. Even if raw products are consumed, there's so much harmful potential in milk, it's not worth some possible good. Would you eat tobacco leaves for their high amino acid content? The human body is remarkably adaptable, but cow's milk simply isn't designed for humans.[5]

The fact is that all green leafy vegetables contain calcium. All nuts (raw) contain calcium. And raw sesame seeds contain more calcium than any other food on earth. Also most fruit contains ample calcium. If you're eating fruits and vegetables daily and some raw nuts even occasionally, you can't have a calcium deficiency. The best sources of calcium are raw sesame seeds, all raw nuts, kelp, dulse, all leafy greens, and concentrated fruits such as figs, dates, and prunes. And if you're still worried, sprinkle some ground raw sesame seeds on your salad or on your vegetables every so often, and you couldn't have a calcium deficiency even if you wanted one. We certainly are not dependent on our bovine friends for calcium. From what does the cow obtain all its calcium? *Grain and*

[5] Herbert M. Shelton, Ph.D. *The Hygienic Care of Children*. Bridgeport, Connecticut: Natural Hygiene Press, 1970.

N. W. Walker, M.D. *Diet and Salad Suggestions*. Phoenix, Arizona: Norwalk Press, 1971.

Hannah Allen. 'Lesson #33, Why We Should Not Eat Animal Products in Any Form.' In *The Life Science Health System*. Austin, Texas: Life Science, 1984.

grass! Cows sure as life don't drink milk or eat cheese for it.

It is important to understand calcium's role in the human body. One of its main functions is to neutralize acid in the system. Many people who think they have a calcium deficiency are on highly acidic diets, so the calcium in their bodies is constantly being usurped to neutralize the acid. They are getting plenty of calcium in their diets, but it is continually used up. **ALL DAIRY PRODUCTS EXCEPT BUTTER ARE EXTREMELY ACID-FORMING.** Butter is a fat and is therefore neutral. Since fat retards the digestion of protein, it is best *not* to eat butter with any protein. Butter *can,* however, be eaten with carbohydrates. The irony is that people are consuming dairy products for calcium, and the existing calcium in their systems is being used to neutralize the effects of the dairy products they are eating. The idea should not be to load up the body with calcium but rather to alter eating habits so that less acid is formed in the system. That way the calcium will be utilized to its fullest potential.

When you are cutting back on dairy consumption, you may notice peeling or brittle nails or minor hair loss. These changes are not to be mistaken for somewhat similar occurrences in very rare instances of protein deficiency. If you *are* concerned, check with your physician. Your body is making the adjustment from the absorption of the coarser calcium found in dairy products to the absorption of the finer calcium found in *raw* nuts, seeds, fruits, and vegetables.

The body will replace fingernails and hair in the same way that sloughed-off skin is replaced. It's difficult to notice, but your skin is regularly sloughing off and being replaced by healthier tissue. In the same way the body will replace lost hair with more lustrous hair, and lost fingernails with stronger, sturdier nails.

Raw nuts are particularly helpful if you do experience a change in your nails or hair. They are incorporated in the program in combination with raw vegetables. Half a cup of raw nuts a day is plenty for the average person. If, when you cut back on dairy products, you immediately take advantage of raw nuts and seeds and have them two or three times a week, your nails and hair will in all likelihood become stronger and more lustrous than ever before.

It has been my experience over the last 15 years that many allergies and breathing problems can be directly tied to dairy consumption – especially asthma. I have personally assisted over two dozen people in eliminating asthma from their lives, and I know of many more people who were helped by other Natural Hygiene practitioners. In *all* cases dairy products were consumed by these individuals. My observations have been similar to those of Beth Snodgrass and Dr Herbert Shelton. The same holds true of children with ear infections. Ear infections are so common that they are actually considered to be a normal part of childhood! Any child who has ever had an ear infection, I would be willing to wager, was either fed dairy products or formula, or both! Kids not fed either dairy products or formula rarely have ear infections. Kids who *are* fed these products do. I know many kids who have never had ear infections, because their parents had the wisdom not to hook their children on these two nonfoods.

I know you've heard experts say dairy products are an important part of a healthy diet. And there *are* experts who say the opposite. To prevent yourself from throwing your hands up in disgust or frustration, make your own decision based on your own resources. Does it *make sense* for humans to be consuming cow's milk?

That's the answer to whether or not you should eat dairy products. Because no matter in what form they are eaten, no matter how tasty they are, if you eat dairy products, you're vicariously suckling from a cow. Does that make sense to *you* or not?

There is one element common to any weight-loss program. Without it, you stack the deck against yourself. That essential ingredient is, of course . . .

CHAPTER 11

Exercise

No weight-loss program concerned with your health is going to work for you without exercise. FIT FOR LIFE is certainly no exception. To guarantee the benefits you deserve from the effort you will put into this program, do some form of aerobics exercise every day. For the body cycles to function effectively, it is imperative to integrate the outlined principles of good eating habits with a well-balanced exercise program. You don't have to exercise yourself into a state of exhaustion; that will only waste energy. But every day you should see to it that your heart is exercised. An aerobics exercise is one that stimulates the respiratory and circulatory systems. This way fresh oxygenated blood reaches all areas of your body, a must if you want your body to operate efficiently. The heart is a muscle, and just like any other muscle, if you don't use it, you lose it. The idea is to do something every day to make yourself pant and sweat. Actually horses sweat, men perspire, and women glow. So get out there and glow and perspire, folks! THIS PROGRAM WILL NOT WORK AS WELL WITHOUT EXERCISE! The benefits extolled in the prior chapters will be severely diminished by depriving the body of the exercise it requires.

There are many aerobic activities to choose from: swimming, tennis, jumping rope, light jogging, bike riding, and brisk walking, as well as aerobics classes. You can also do some stretching and weight lifting if you wish, but the aerobics part is imperative.

Many people are now choosing to own some kind of aerobics equipment that they can use in their own homes. There are reasonably priced exercise bikes, rowing machines, rebounders (minitrampolines), and many other excellent pieces of exercise equipment now being manufactured for home use. If your time is precious (and whose isn't?), and you can't always make it to the gym, consider owning some form of aerobics exerciser that you can use whenever you have the time.

Look into rebounding. It is a terrific way to insure yourself an excellent full-body workout every day. You can own one of these reasonably priced mini-trampolines and jump on it right after you get out of bed in the morning. No special attire necessary. No distances to travel. This is the workout that astronauts and sports teams have been using for years – and you can do it in the comfort of your own home (or better yet, out in the fresh air, in your own garden). Rebounding is a terrific aerobics exercise that people of all ages can enjoy, without the risks to the bone structure that come from jogging on pavement, or to the lower back from strenuous aerobic calisthenics. It strengthens and tones every cell of the body because it works against the gravitational pull.

There is a minimum of aerobics exercise that should be performed every day. That minimum is a 20-minute *brisk* walk. This is truly a minimum. More would be great, but if you walk briskly for at least twenty minutes, you will be performing enough aerobics to facilitate the working of this program. The ideal time to do this exercise, or any exercise, is early in the morning. The air is freshest then, and so is your body. There are physical benefits from early morning exercise because your body is most capable of utilizing exercise at that time, but also there are tremendous psychological benefits. I think that anyone interested in losing weight or generally improving his or her wellbeing knows deep down the importance of exercise. Unfortunately for some it's so easy to find a reason not to exercise. Knowing one *should* exercise regularly but not doing it can create negative feelings toward oneself, and that is an energy drain. The way this happens is every time you think of exercise, all day, if you haven't done any yet, you say to yourself, 'Well, I haven't done any yet today, and I probably won't be able to later, so I'll do it tomorrow.' Meanwhile you can't help feeling guilty. However, if you exercise first thing in the morning, then every time you think of exercise during the day, it's with a feeling like 'Yeah! I've already exercised!' It fills you with a fantastic positive feeling for yourself, and these feelings spill over into other areas of your life. Everything is enhanced. Once you get into the habit of exercising every morning, you'll get to the point where you'll actually feel disappointed if you miss a day.

In my own case I had the overweight person's typical resistance to exercise, so I had to regiment myself to exercise every morning. Some days I would wake up with thoughts like Boy, I've been so good, I'll just take a well-deserved day off. Or Hey, even some pros say you should take a day off once in a while. But while I was saying these things to myself, which was just the old fat me, Blimpo, trying to hold on to the past, I would be putting on my exercise clothes and preparing myself to work out. Even as I would climb onto my bike for my regular 10-mile routine, a part of me was trying to talk myself out of it. But the new me, the one that liked being slim and wanted to stay that way, won out, and now I look forward with anticipation to my morning constitutional. The real benefits became apparent to me one month after I started. When I first started exercising regularly, my resting heartbeat was 72 beats per minute. One month later it was 54! In one month I had strengthened and improved the function of my heart by 18 beats per minute. That's over 15,000 fewer beats per day! This translates to millions fewer beats a year. We're talking about longevity. Lessening the burden on the heart by several million beats a year can't help but lengthen one's life. That's exciting! Not only has exercise become fun for me, it has afforded me enormous benefits.

I am certain without even a vestige of doubt that the addition of regular exercise to my improved eating is a major contributing factor to being able to keep my weight down where I want it.

PLEASE DON'T MAKE THE MISTAKE OF EXCLUDING EXERCISE FROM YOUR DAILY LIFE. THE SUCCESS OF THIS PROGRAM DEPENDS ON IT.

There are few people indeed who could not at least take a brisk walk. Just as the principles of eating should be a part of your new life-style, exercise, too, must play an important role.

While I'm talking about your new life-style, a couple of other quick items deserve attention: fresh air and sunshine. Few people realize how much nourishment our bodies obtain from the air we breathe. Fresh, clean air is a most valuable life force, along with sunshine, which is the source of all life on this planet. Make a point of supplying yourself with both of these important elements of health as often as you can. They will accelerate your progress in losing weight.

A walk in the woods or at the seashore, or a hike in the country, will do wonders for your physical well-being and your emotional and spiritual outlook. Most important, it is essential to have a window open when you sleep. Even if you must add an extra blanket for warmth, fresh air circulating while you sleep is invaluable. The body can be more effective during the assimilation and elimination cycles if it is given fresh air while it works and is not forced to breathe air that is laden with toxins it has just eliminated.

There is wrong information going around today that causes many of us in the health field to cringe. That is the *unbelieveable misconception* that the sun is dangerous! THE SUN IS THE SOURCE OF ALL LIFE ON THIS PLANET! THIS IS A TRUTH THAT MUST NEVER BE FORGOTTEN! Without the sun there is no life as we know it! We create valuable nutrients with the help of sunlight. It is also a great assistant in detoxification and weight loss, since it opens our pores and allows toxins to exit through the skin. *Anything* that's abused can be dangerous. If you hold your head under water, you'll drown. Does that mean we should not use water? Obviously the potential for danger is there. However, it doesn't mean that we should avoid it. There is also a potential for danger with the sun. *Too much* can burn you, just as too much water can drown you. But we are not talking about abuse. DO NOT AVOID THE SUN! TAKE ADVANTAGE OF IT! Tanning lotions and sunscreens are not recommended. It is far better to build one's tolerance to the sun slowly than to use oils, screens, or lotions that prevent absorption of all the ultraviolet and infrared rays. They also inhibit the workings of the oil-secreting glands. The important point to remember is that it is not merely a tan that we get from the sun, but a revitalizing of our entire bodies – not limited to the skin. If you do use oils or lotions, avoid those containing chemicals. If you can, take a half-hour in the sun every day or as often as possible, preferably in the morning. This is absolutely essential if you wish to have that golden glow that is so much a part of living the **HIGH-ENERGY LIFE-STYLE.**

Most assuredly, physical exercise, fresh air, and sunlight play a crucial role in the attainment of well-being. There is another exceptional tool at your disposal that can dramatically improve every aspect of your health. It is something you *already possess,* and you need only to start to use it to reap its many rewards. It is a phenomenon that emanates from the belief that . . .

CHAPTER 12

You Are What You Think You Are

It may seem as if we have no conscious control over our bodies' condition, because we are generally taught that there is little connection between our thoughts and our physical bodies. Whether or not this is the case, certainly a positive outlook toward oneself doesn't hurt. It is my personal belief, and there are others who share it, that we can actually assist the body's quest for health with our thoughts. In his highly acclaimed best-selling book *Anatomy of an Illness,* Dr Norman Cousins attributed his recovery largely to the positive manner in which he viewed his situation. *Beyond the Relaxation Response* by Dr Herbert Benson, head of behavioral medicine at Boston's Beth Israel Hospital and professor of cardiology at Harvard, presents a strong case for the mind's power to change the body physically.

I spoke earlier of the incalculable wisdom and flawless accuracy of the human organism. Also discussed was the tremendous role our beliefs play in our lives. If you truly believe you can do something, **YOU CAN**!

Every cell in your body is teeming with life and

possesses its own intelligence. Each cell is like a soldier in the army, awaiting its instructions. We are constantly sending messages or commands to our cells, and those commands are carried out diligently. What I'm suggesting is that we can consciously direct our cells to do what we want them to do. The body will bring about whatever result the conscious mind desires. The mind is continuously assessing the body's condition and forming images in line with what it believes to be true. We can literally change our bodies by changing the way we think about them, even in the face of data or evidence that conflicts.

We are constantly sending ourselves a barrage of suggestions about our weight and our health. These can be either positive or negative suggestions – helpful or harmful. We have at our disposal the means to assist our bodies in losing weight and upgrading our health, but to *be* healthy we must start to *believe* we are healthy! To lose weight, start by believing that you CAN and WILL! Your cells are awaiting your instructions.

For example, if you look in the mirror and say to yourself, 'Gosh, I'm fat,' mentally you are sending messages that automatically affect your body in just that way. They are commands to the cellular structure to keep you overweight. To tell yourself over and over again that you have fat or unsightly thighs serves only to instruct them to remain so. But what is simply marvelous is that your cells will automatically obey your *last* instruction. So even if you have had a negative self-image for years and have habitually sent negative messages to yourself as a matter of course, you can, *this very moment,* start to reverse that trend. If, because of habit, you say something negative about yourself, merely acknowledge it, but do not reinforce it. Instead, simply suggest that the remedy be carried out positively. If you should say, 'Boy, look at that flabby stomach,' immediately counteract that statement with a more useful one: 'I'm losing weight from my mid-section,' or 'My thighs are getting smaller,' or 'I AM LOSING WEIGHT!' Your body will reflect those positive suggestions, which will supersede the negative ones. You will in effect be giving your body *permission* to lose weight! This is a tool that works, and you can employ it as often as you wish.

Upgrading your diet by employing the principles laid out, exercising daily to supply fresh oxygenated blood to your cells, and sending a flow of positive suggestions to reinforce the success you are seeking form a winning combination that simply can't be beaten.

The greatest thinkers the world has ever known, from Da Vinci to Einstein to Mark Twain, have always agreed that when it comes to understanding any given subject, what we know is but an infinitesimal speck of what there is to know. Statements like 'The more we learn, the more there is to learn,' and 'The more we know, the more we realize how much we don't know' indicate that the tremendous body of knowledge that makes up the great unknown will always be bringing new information to light. The enormity of what is yet to be learned about the human body and how it operates is unfathomable.

Some people's *beliefs* may prevent them from accepting that they can consciously direct the shape of their bodies. But it is in the best interest of anyone who is looking to lose weight and improve health to employ whatever measures are available that can potentially lend help. From a common-sense point of view, doesn't it seem as if sending a constant flow of positive suggestions to yourself would be useful?

Once again, this tool, like all the others presented

in this book, is an idea for you to investigate. Try it and see if it works for you. I think you are going to be pleasantly surprised.

Now that all the principles have been covered, this is a good time to answer . . .

CHAPTER 13

The Most Frequently Asked Questions

You probably have some specific questions you want answered. The purpose of this chapter is to answer some of the most often asked questions about FIT FOR LIFE.

Q. *Where does drinking coffee or tea fit into this approach to eating?*

A. The fact that less than 9 per cent of the population of this country drink neither coffee nor tea is a clear indication of how prevalent this habit is. About half the people in the United States drink two to three cups a day of these beverages, and another quarter of the population drink six or more cups every day. That means over *two hundred billion* doses of the drug caffeine are consumed every year. Most people would not think of their morning cup of coffee or afternoon tea as a drug. Yet caffeine is addictive, causing withdrawal symptoms when discontinued and inducing both psychological and physical dependence. It certainly sounds like a drug. Caffeine is a stimulant of the central nervous system, similar to cocaine, and has been linked to a host of maladies, including increased heart rate, change in blood vessel diameter, irregular coronary circulation, increased blood pressure, birth defects, diabetes, kidney failure, gastric ulcers, cancer of the pancreas, ringing in the ears, trembling of muscles, restlessness, disturbed sleep, and gastrointestinal irritation. It also upsets the blood sugar level, as it forces the pancreas to secrete insulin.

You may ask if decaffeinated coffee or tea is better. Let me address that with this question: Would you rather fracture your arm or your leg? The decaffeinating process usually requires a highly caustic chemical solvent that permeates the bean, which you ingest. It takes *one* cup of coffee or tea 24 hours to pass through the kidneys and urinary tract. More than one cup in a 24-hour period places an extremely heavy burden on these organs. If you are one of those who drink seven or eight cups of coffee or tea a day, give serious consideration to owning your own dialysis machine. Most certainly coffee decaffeinated with water or non-chemical methods is better than the chemically decaffeinated, but that should not give license to drinking it. It is still acid-forming – that's the problem.

Coffee consumed with food forces the food to leave the stomach prematurely and also slows down the motility of the intestines. Undigested food in a slowly functioning intestinal tract is a major contributor to constipation. The caustic effect of coffee is what causes the intestines to move food through rapidly for some people. The coffee itself takes 24 hours to be processed out through the kidneys.

The extreme importance of avoiding acid-forming foods in the diet has been stressed throughout this book. The human body has a pH balance, which reflects the degree of acidity or alkalinity. The pH levels can fall between zero and 14, with zero totally acid, 14 totally alkaline, and 7 neutral. The blood is slightly alkaline, with a pH of 7.35 to 7.40. If a person's blood were to reach even the neutral level of 7.0, that person would be in great danger. The leeway between 7.35 and 7.40 is small; there is very little leeway before the blood is thrown out of balance. Coffee and tea happen to be pure acid in the body. The more acid in the blood, the more the body will retain water in an attempt to neutralize it. This adds weight to your body.

All of this is not presented in an attempt to scare you into giving up coffee and tea, but rather to help you become more aware of what effect they have on the body's health and to what extent they either assist or prevent successful weight loss.

Some people can simply quit drinking these beverages at once; others have to 'wean' themselves from them slowly. Some people have been drinking just one cup in the morning for years and don't want to give it up.[1] All are okay. Certainly one cup of coffee a day is not going to make or break this program. Obviously no coffee or tea in your diet is best, but if you can at least cut down, then do so. The better you feel, the better you will want to feel, and you will naturally do what is necessary to bring about that feeling of well-being as you progress. Incidentally, if you do want to have a hot beverage other than coffee or tea once in a while, try some of the herbal teas, particularly those preparations from Celestial Seasonings. They have good flavors and most are naturally caffeine-free.

What is most important is direction. Keep in mind your goal of a slim, healthy body and make regular

[1] If it is simply a *hot* drink you want in the morning, try hot water and lemon juice. This is a satisfying beverage and the lemon, unlike other fruits, contains no sugar and will not ferment in the hot water.

strides in that direction. You are on a journey; let it be fun, not an ordeal. You can drive from the West Coast to the East Coast in three days at breakneck speed and miss all the sights and splendor this country has to offer, or you can take three weeks and enjoy yourself. Take your time, and be confident that you will reach your destination a happier, healthier person for the effort expended on your own behalf.

Q. *What about sodas?*

A. Over two hundred million soft drinks are consumed in this country each year. Actually they are anything but soft on your body, except for your teeth. Dr Clive McCay of Cornell University showed that soft drinks can completely erode tooth enamel and make teeth as soft as mush within two days (as described in *The Poisoned Needle* by Eleanor McBean). The ingredient that is the culprit here is a horrific concoction called phosphoric acid. These drinks also contain malic acid, carbonic acid, and erythorbic acid, among other things. The malic and citric acids to be found naturally in fruits and vegetables are of a nature that turns alkaline in the system. The ones to be found in soft drinks remain acid because they are fractionated and usually extracted with heat. Your pH balance can be thrown into turmoil just by reading the label of a soft drink! There are several other harmful ingredients to be found in these drinks as well, plus refined white sugar, about five teaspoons per 8-ounce serving. The only difference between regular and diet sodas is that instead of sugar a substitute is used, so harmful that each container has to have a warning on the label just like cigarettes. Plus most sodas have our old nemesis, caffeine. Some of the additives used are coal-tar derivatives, another carcinogen. When soft drinks are taken with food, it leads to fermentation instead of good digestion. Aside from tricking your body into thinking they taste good, there are no benefits in sodas.

It's criminal that such a lethal beverage is so routinely given to our children. The caffeine should be reason enough not to give it to children. It's interesting that most parents won't allow their children to drink coffee, but they condone caffeinated soft drinks. You may be wondering why caffeine is added to these drinks. According to Dr Royal Lee of the Foundation for Nutritional Research, 'Cola is loaded with habit-forming caffeine so that once the victim becomes accustomed to the stimulant, he cannot very well get along without it. There is only one reason for putting caffeine in a soft drink – to make it habit-forming.' Here again, direction is what is of primary concern. If you can cut down on this nonnutritious, empty-caloried conglomeration of acids and cancer-causing chemicals, by all means do. There are many carbonated waters on the market that although not ideal (because of the high salt content and inorganic minerals) are far better than 'soft' drinks.[2]

Q. *Is a little chocolate now and again all that bad?*

A. A *little bit* of almost anything now and again is not that bad. There are, however, a couple of ingredients in chocolate that are not positive contributors to health. The first, and this may start to sound like a crusade, is a caffeine-related substance called theobromine. According to Dr Bruce Ames of the University of California, Berkeley, theobromine gives power to

[2] Canada Dry's salt-free seltzer water with lemon or lime is an excellent substitute.

certain carcinogens in human cells that damage DNA. It also causes testicular atrophy. The other ingredient can really put a damper on a weight-loss program: refined white sugar. In the process of refining sugar, every vestige of life and nutrient is stripped from it. All the fiber, vitamins, minerals, everything is virtually removed, leaving only a deadly remnant. Sugar makes people fat because it supplies only empty, low-quality calories and excessive carbohydrates that are converted to fat. This causes you to overeat to obtain needed nutrients. When you eat foods high in sugar, the body must have additional food to get the nutrients it needs. This tends to add weight. The practice that will help eliminate that craving for sweets more than anything else is the *correct* consumption of fruit. The sugar in fruit is untampered with and supplies the body with the nutrients it craves. Plus, because it supplies fiber and bulk, it satisfies, whereas refined sugar is fiber-free, and even after eating quite a bit of it you can still feel empty. Refined sugar eaten in any shape or form – in food, in candy, or in liquids – ferments in the system, causing the formation of acetic acid, carbonic acid, and alcohol. The process of refining sugar causes the sugar's fermentation in the body.

It's difficult to show how any one particular type of food adversely affects an overall eating plan. Taken out of context, it tends to seem less serious than it actually may be. But coupled with other negative influences, it contributes to the eventual breakdown of the body. Picture a large bay window. If you were to throw a small pebble at the window, it would not break. But throw 100,000 small pebbles, and the window will shatter. Each negative influence on your body is like one pebble, and all together those influences can and will break down your body's health. The fewer pebbles you throw at the window, the less likely the window is to break. The fewer negative influences the body has to contend with, whether they are coffee, tea, soda, alcohol, or candy, the less likely the body is to remain overweight. Even just *cutting down* is beneficial; it's fewer pebbles.

Q. *I've heard that a little wine with a meal helps to digest the food. Is this true?*

A. Whoever is responsible for that bit of tomfoolery surely sits on the board of one of the major wineries. The body no more needs help to digest food than it needs help to blink its eyes or to breathe. All are autonomic responses. Digestion simply takes place when food is in the stomach. If anything, wine *retards* the digestion of food. In the same way your motor responses are slowed down when under the influence of alcohol, digestion is also slowed down.

Wine is fermented, which causes any food it comes into contact with to spoil. All alcohol places a heavy burden on the kidneys and liver. If you enjoy wine, try to drink it on an empty stomach. It will take less to 'loosen you up,' and it won't spoil any food. Moderation is the key. Remember, the fewer pebbles against the window, the better.

Q. *It seems that on this type of diet I wouldn't need to take any vitamin and mineral supplements. Is that true?*

A. Absolutely! The controversy of whether or not supplements are necessary could fill a book of its own. How did we manage for centuries without them? The manufacture and sale of these supplements is one of the ten largest businesses in the United States. Supplement sales now generate 2 billion dollars a year! I wonder to what extent some of the claims one hears are commercially motivated.

In terms of your health there is a long list of experts in the field of nutrition, both inside and outside the medical community, who are expressing grave concerns over the health threat emerging from taking vitamin and mineral supplements. Dr. Myron Winick, the director of the Institute of Human Nutrition at Columbia University, indicates that some old standby vitamins long considered totally innocuous are producing medical problems, including nerve damage, mild intestinal distress, and fatal liver damage (reported in the *Los Angeles Times,* 20 December 1983).

Our actual need for vitamins and minerals has been grossly exaggerated. The amount of vitamins necessary for the human body for a *full year* would not even fill a thimble. And that is the RDA (recommended daily allowance), which is *twice* what our actual needs are. These statements may sound shocking, but they are the facts. Every vitamin and mineral necessary for your body can be found in abundance in fruits and vegetables. The body has such a small requirement for these elements that even if you ate only a small amount of *fresh* fruits and vegetables, you would be meeting your requirements. This program is designed to incorporate into your diet more than ample amounts of what you need, in their purest, most easily absorbable form. *Nothing* is of the quality that is found in fruits and vegetables, notwithstanding some of the advertising claims boasting that their product is 100 per cent natural. Being 100 per cent natural would mean as it was created by nature. I personally have never seen a vitamin or mineral pill tree.

Man-made supplements are simply not what was intended for the human body. In the process of extracting and fractionating elements, they are rendered worthless. Vitamin supplements become toxic in the body.[3] The body can most efficiently use vitamins and minerals that are consumed along with all the other constituents of any given food. Once removed and isolated, vitamins lose their value. And synthesized vitamins are virtually worthless. Right now technology exists that can create a grain of wheat in the laboratory. Every chemical component can be duplicated and made into a grain of wheat. But if it's put into the ground, it won't grow. Yet grains of wheat taken from tombs that are 4,000 years old will sprout if put into the ground! There is a very subtle ingredient missing in the synthesized wheat: life force! This same ingredient is also missing in synthesized vitamins and minerals. Worse than being worthless, these products are treated as toxic waste in the body. Our goal is always to *eliminate* toxic waste, not produce more.

The body also has what is called the law of minimum. In other words, once the vitamin and mineral requirements are met, any more must be eliminated as excess. If you had a small glass and a pitcher full of juice, you could fill the glass only to the brim. If you continue to pour, you will only waste the juice as it overflows the glass. That is precisely how it works when there are more vitamins and minerals in the body than it has a need for. Again the excess is treated as toxic waste and usurps your precious energy as the body tries to rid itself of it. This places a heavy burden on the liver and the kidneys in the process. When you take supplements, they will *always* be in excess unless you are

[3] Robert McCarter, Ph.D., and Elizabeth McCarter, Ph.D. 'A Statement on Vitamins,' 'Vitamins and Cures,' and 'Other Unnecessary Supplements.' *Health Reporter* 11 (1984): 10, 24.

on the most devitalized, processed, denatured diet imaginable. The eating life-style laid out in FIT FOR LIFE is most assuredly brimming over with all the vitamins and minerals you will need. Health has to be earned. Health is produced by healthful living. It can't be purchased in a bottle. So, save your energy . . . and your money.

Q. *Just how harmful is table salt?*

A. The Egyptians used salt for embalming. Let's take the hint! This year Americans will consume 500 million pounds of salt. That's a lot of embalming. Salt is everywhere and in everything from pet food to baby food. Salt is a major contributing factor to the increasing incidence of hypertension, or high blood pressure, in this country. It is so caustic to the sensitive inner tissues of the body that water is retained to neutralize its acidic effect. This adds weight to the body. Overuse of salt can contribute to a severe affliction of the kidneys called nephritis.

When you consider that many people consume coffee, tea, soda pop, alcohol, supplements, and salt every day, all of which must be excreted by the kidneys, it is no small wonder why so many people die annually from kidney failure. Whatever we can do to save our poor overworked kidneys should be done. Salt should be used sparingly, if at all. For those who wish to continue using salt, Dr N. W. Walker recommends coarse ground sea salt, which is less processed than regular salt. Coarse ground sea salt can be used in a salt grinder. There are also many seasoned salts and salt-free seasonings (see the Shopping List, page 200) that can help cut down on salt intake.

Q. *Why does it seem as if so many people today either have hypoglycemia or think they do? And doesn't eating fruit aggravate a hypoglycemic condition?*

A. The reason that so many people have hypoglycemia and that so many others think they do is twofold. First, the range of possible symptoms of hypoglycemia is so extensive that it would be surprising if there were anyone without at least one of the symptoms. The list of *62* possible symptoms includes emotional upsets, moodiness, stuffy nose, fatigue, exhaustion, confusion, inability to think straight, anxiety, irritability, and inability to decide easily. It even includes gas, indigestion, flatulence, and feeling *sleepy after meals*! Wow! There probably aren't three people in the United States who haven't experienced at least one of *those* symptoms, and there are about 45 more! Second, the Standard American Diet (SAD) is such that its energy-usurping, acid-producing nature is certainly consistent with creating low blood sugar, which is another term for hypoglycemia.

In the chapter on the correct consumption of fruit, it was stated that fruit has borne the brunt of more unjustifiable criticism than any other food. The second part of your question is a classic example of the almost universal misunderstanding of fruit's ever-so-important role in acquiring and maintaining a high level of health. As odd as it may seem, fruit is actually what will most effectively and efficiently overcome the problem of hypoglycemia. I don't mean it will effectively suppress the symptoms; I mean it will *remove the cause* so the symptoms never appear. The most common means of suppressing symptoms is by eating, usually something very heavy like protein food such as meat or eggs. This will cause the symptoms to abate by diverting the energy that was causing the symptoms to the stomach to digest the food. It is a temporary measure that insures the prolonged existence of the problem, leading to more frequent eating. There is a far more rational approach that can eliminate the frequent meals *and* the hypoglycemia.

What exactly is low blood sugar? It was pointed out earlier that the number-one prerequisite of a food should be its fuel value. That approximately 90 per cent of our food should supply us with the glucose needed to carry out life's functions. The brain uses only one fuel: sugar in the form of glucose. It does not use fat or protein or anything but glucose, which is taken from the bloodstream to meet the brain's requirements. If there is not a sufficient amount of utilizable sugar in the blood to satisfy the needs of the brain, an alarm goes off. This alarm manifests itself as the symptoms of hypoglycemia. So the problem boils down to not having enough sugar in the blood. To rectify this situation, simply add sugar to the blood. It's extremely hard to have low blood sugar if you have plenty of sugar in the blood. Here's where the confusion usually appears. It is absolutely, positively imperative that the *right kind of sugar* be introduced into the bloodstream. Any kind of *processed* sugar will only make the situation worse. The kind of sugar that will do the job is the sugar found in fresh fruit! In the fruit it's called fructose; inside the body it turns to glucose faster than any other carbohydrate. What is essential to remember is that the fruit must be eaten *correctly.* This means on an *empty* stomach. Because the sugar is in its natural, organic state, it will pass swiftly through the stomach and be in the bloodstream within an hour.

By following the program in Part Two you will automatically be eating fruit correctly, which will help you eliminate the *cause* of hypoglycemia. For many people who have suffered from hypoglycemia for years without relief, this explanation may sound overly simplified. But we have many case histories of people with long-standing hypoglycemia. Many had confirmed its existence with the Glucose Tolerance Test and subsequently eliminated the problem successfully by employing the FIT FOR LIFE technique.

Q. *Is it all right for a woman to go on the program during her pregnancy?* (This is a perfect question for Marilyn to answer.)

A. Yes, *but* preparation for a healthy child should begin *before* conception, at least six months or longer, if possible. Given the nature of diet's importance during pregnancy, consultation with your doctor about dietary changes is advised. However, during pregnancy it is never too late to *gradually* upgrade one's diet. Whatever changes of a positive nature are made can only improve the condition of mother and child and allow for an easier delivery.

The program fulfills all the dietary requirements for both mother and child during gestation. Because of the ample fresh fruit recommended, the primary requirement – abundant fuel in the form of glucose – is satisfied. Many of the ingredients in the daily raw salads further help fulfill the glucose requirement, and these salads provide the mother and baby with the minerals and vitamins necessary for proper growth and development. Actually the most beneficial diet during pregnancy (and at any other time!) is a diet that has a preponderance of raw fruits and vegetables, and some raw nuts and seeds. This will supply all the fuel, amino acids, minerals, fatty acids, and vitamins needed to perpetuate a high level of health. This program is more than adequate in fulfilling these requirements. That foods are combined properly insures that maximum nutrients will be available for absorption at each meal with a minimum of waste. *Proper* diet will insure an energetic, delightful pregnancy. *Improper* diet can turn this inspiring experience into an ordeal.

Frequently, pregnant women are advised to drink plenty of pasteurized milk to insure that they get enough calcium for their babies' teeth and bones. The truth is most adults do not have the digestive enzymes lactase and renin that are necessary to get calcium from milk, for it is bound in the *indigestible* protein complement casein. In addition, pasteurization causes the calcium to be unusable due to heat derangement.[4] To insure that they are getting adequate *usable* calcium, pregnant women should remember it is readily available in abundance in fresh fruit, beans, cauliflower, cabbage, lettuce and other leafy greens, nuts and seeds (almonds and sesame seeds particularly), asparagus, and figs.[5] *Fresh* orange juice helps the body to retain calcium, according to Dr Herbert Shelton in *The Hygienic Care of Children.* Adequate sunshine is also required for calcium metabolism. The fetus stores a calcium supply in its tissues, which it draws upon during the later stages of pregnancy, so it is most crucial

[4] There are several Hygienic authorities on the subject of utilizing calcium from pasteurized cow's milk. All say the same thing: We can't!

Herbert M. Shelton, Ph.D. *The Hygienic Care of Children.* Bridgeport, Connecticut: Natural Hygiene Press, 1970.

N. W. Walker, M.D. *Diet and Salad Suggestions.* Phoenix, Arizona: Norwalk Press, 1971.

Robin A. Hur. *Food Reform: Our Desperate Need.* Austin, Texas: Heidelburg, 1975.

Joyce M. Kling. 'Lesson #55, Prenatal Care for Better Infant and Maternal Health and Less Painful Childbirth.' In *The Life Science Health System,* by T. C. Fry. Austin, Texas: Life Science, 1984.

M. Bircher-Benner. *Eating Your Way to Health.* Baltimore: Penguin Books, 1973.

[5] See Day Sixteen of the Program for Fresh Almond Milk, page 300.

for the pregnant woman to obtain and retain adequate calcium for herself and her child during the *early* months of pregnancy.

Pregnant women are also counseled to drink milk so they will have a rich milk supply for the baby. That is ludicrous. Do cows enrich *their* milk supply by drinking the milk of another species? Of course they don't! They eat lots of grain and grass. We, like all other mammals, *automatically* make milk when we are pregnant. The consumption of lots of fresh fruit and fresh green vegetables makes our milk even more rich and abundant. By the way, if you are given folic acid pills 'for your milk,' you might want to substitute a daily green salad, which is a fine, readily available *natural* source of folic acid.

Remember, it is not *how much* calcium is contained in the foods one eats, but how much is actually *usable* (absorbed and retained). The taking of dolomite or calcium supplements during pregnancy *does not* provide *usable* calcium, and frequently causes harmful calcium deposits in the placenta. These supplements provide an *inorganic* calcium (whether or not they are labeled organic), which our bodies simply cannot use.

Dr Ralph C. Cinque has conducted extensive experimentation and research on this subject. The information here is taken directly from text material he wrote.[6] Again we are dealing with a difference in philosophies. Natural Hygiene is diametrically opposed to the acquisition of vitamins and minerals

[6] Ralph C. Cinque, Ph.D. 'Lesson #55, Prenatal Care for Better Infant and Maternal Health and Less Painful Childbirth.' In *The Life Science Health System,* by T. C. Fry. Austin, Texas: Life Science, 1984.
Rose Dosti. 'Nutritional Needs Greater for Pregnant Teen-agers, Over 30s.' *Los Angeles Times,* 31 May 1984.
'Vitamin Megadoses Can Be Harmful.' *Los Angeles Times,* 20 December 1983.

from sources other than natural ones, *natural* meaning gardens and orchards, not pills. I'm sure supporters of both sides of this issue could knock heads and be very convincing for their own philosophies. The fact remains that, according to Natural Hygiene,which *this* book is all about, all vitamin and mineral supplements, because they are fractionated, are treated as toxic waste in the body. As in so many other issues concerning nutrition, some traditional doctors are beginning to recognize the Hygienic viewpoint. Dr Vicki G. Hufnagel, speaking at the Fourteenth Annual Nutrition Conference sponsored by the Dairy Council of California, said, 'We are just learning what harm they can do to a small embryo. Vitamins are drugs.' Dr Hufnagel is an obstetrician/gynecologist. Dr Myron Winick, Director of the Institute of Human Nutrition at Columbia University, stated, 'Some people treat vitamin pills like candy, but they're not. They're more like drugs. And we all know that there are no safe drugs, only safe doses.'

Far better than taking manufactured dolomite would be to sprinkle the mineral dolomite (like lime) in your garden, and then grow leafy green lettuce that will provide you with plenty of *usable organic* calcium! It is imperative to understand that calcium deficiencies are the result not only of taking in insufficient amounts of calcium, but also from overeating and miscombining foods, practices that seriously impair digestion and absorption. Pregnancy does not carry with it the license to overeat! A weight gain of more than twenty to twenty-five pounds can result in an oversize baby and a high-risk delivery.[7] Pregnant women tend to overeat

[7] In my last pregnancy I gained a total of only 14 pounds and both the baby and I were in excellent health. One hour after the birth, I was up bathing him – with an abundance of energy!

when they are eating highly processed, adulterated foods. They are overeating in response to their bodies' signals that nutritional needs are not being met. FIT FOR LIFE emphasizes the foods that are the most nourishing for mother and child and will actually help you to keep your weight gain down.

Incidentally, during pregnancy more than any other time, certain items are harmful. This program will help you gradually eliminate many of them. The placenta, which is supposed to filter out harmful substances ingested by the mother and protect the fetus from these substances, has *no* effectiveness in screening drugs, alcohol, tobacco poisons, caffeine, salt, vinegar, and chemical additives and preservatives in processed foods. By following the program you will automatically be eliminating these harmful influences. None of them are included in any of the menu items, with the exception of salt, which is always indicated as an *optional* ingredient. As far as the other, more harmful substances, let's be candid for the sake of our future children. There is no 'safe' drug, prescription or nonprescription, that can be taken during pregnancy, notwithstanding the fact that many pregnant women are still being counseled to take drugs. Thalidomide was merely the tip of the iceberg. *All* drugs, from aspirin to pain relievers to tranquilizers, carry with them the risk of deformity and mental retardation for your baby. Alcohol consumption during pregnancy can result in 'fetal alcohol syndrome,' a deformity of the face and head that is frequently accompanied by mental retardation. Caffeine in coffee, tea, sodas, chocolate, and many drugs has been linked to birth defects. Cigarette smoking causes oxygen deprivation to the fetus, resulting in premature, low-weight births and mental retardation.

Obviously, none of these harmful substances are

advocated in the program. My reason for discussing them here is to heighten the awareness among pregnant women of what their effects can be on the unborn child. In 12 per cent or more of all births in our country defects now occur, and this number is increasing every year as more and more chemicals and poisons enter our environment and our diet.

Being pregnant is a special time requiring more than any other time a special consciousness about the body's needs. Following the program will help insure the right food and the fresh air and sunshine that are integral factors to a healthy pregnancy. Plenty of rest and regular exercise are also necessary.

Sometimes individuals have special requirements. All changes in diet during pregnancy should be made *gradually* and under the supervision of your midwife, health adviser, or doctor.

This concludes Part I, in which I have endeavored to give you a clear understanding of *what* changes in life-style are necessary for you to overcome your weight problem once and for all, and *why* you would want to make these changes. In Part II Marilyn will give you some important hints on *how* to make these changes so that your new life-style will be a lasting one. Drawing from her understanding of American dietary addictions, from her background as a creative teacher of gourmet home cooking, and from her solid grasp of the Natural Hygiene principles, she has outlined a four-week program that will show you how to prepare a variety of delicious, properly combined, high-water-content meals. The program has been designed to speed you toward your goal of weight loss while comfortably initiating the all-important detoxification of your body.

An effective **WEIGHT LOSS AND HIGH-ENERGY LIFE-STYLE** is now only one meal away, so let's turn over a new leaf in our lives by turning the page to begin . . .

PART II

The Program

By
Marilyn Diamond

Introduction

When I first consulted Harvey in his capacity as a nutritional counselor in 1975, I was going through the most critical health crisis of my life. I came to him in a very discouraged frame of mind. I had a strong medical background[1] and a long history of medical treatment, but for as long as I could remember, I had never really felt *well.* Excess weight was not my *major* concern at that time, although I'm not saying it wasn't *one* of my concerns. I must confess, though, from my early teens I had not been happy with the shape of my body, and since that time I had always worn high heels to achieve a thinner look.

My real problem, although I did not know it at the

[1] During my childhood my father was a biochemist at the National Institutes of Health in Bethesda, Maryland. He subsequently held positions as department head of Microbiology and Molecular Biology at New York University Medical School and Albert Einstein College of Medicine. He is presently the dean of the Graduate School of Medicine at Cornell University.

The medical and scientific professions have an all-encompassing life-style in which I was very much involved as my father's child. I worked in his laboratory during summer vacations, and under his influence I studied biology and chemistry in college.

time, was that I was totally out of energy. I felt terrible, and I was having a great deal of trouble coping with my life. Actually what I was experiencing was not an uncommon phenomenon. Conditions of negative energy are the basis of many of the physical, psychological, and emotional problems being experienced by men, women, *and* children in this country. My symptoms were not unusual: stomach pain, embarrassing skin eruptions, depression, confusion, sudden mood swings, and emotional outbursts. What frightened me was that they were becoming progressively worse. After having been so highly motivated in college that I had been Phi Beta Kappa and magna cum laude, at the age of 31, with two small children, I spent much of my time in depression and tears, wondering how I was ever going to feel well enough to get on with my life. No amount of drugs, treatment, or therapy that I had had over the years had done anything to change or improve my situation. In all the time that I had been medicated for a nervous stomach and debilitated digestive tract, been tranquilized for nervous tension, taken injection therapy for pain, and theorized with the 'experts' about my physical, mental, and emotional 'dis-ease,' no one ever asked me what I was eating! Harvey *did!*

Natural Hygiene, as Harvey was teaching it, supplied me with answers about my health that I had all but given up on finding. What did I learn? Everything I needed to know to help myself feel well! I learned that I was in pain and out of energy because for most of my life I had been overtaxing my system with the *wrong kinds of foods.* Because for so many decades in this country breast-feeding had not been in vogue, I had been among the millions of babies who *never* received breast milk, the *only* food naturally intended for and suitable to the young of the human species. In his most recent book, *How to Raise a Healthy Child in Spite of*

Your Doctor, Dr Robert S. Mendelsohn writes, 'Breast-feeding lays the foundation for healthy physical and emotional growth . . . *Mother's milk, time-tested for millions of years, is the best nutrient for babies because it is nature's perfect food.*'[2]

How did we in our society arrive at that place of ignorance where we actually didn't know what a difference breast-feeding would make in the future health of our children? Dr Mendelsohn places the blame firmly with the commercially motivated formula manufacturers and the pediatricians who help them sell their formulas. He faults obstetricians and pediatricians for failing to emphasize strongly enough the importance of breast-feeding. As a result, millions of children in our society have been and continue to be raised on formula and cow's milk, which are overladen with protein and which some researchers feel contain a coarser and therefore less absorbable calcium than that found in mother's milk. In my case, this led to a highly acidic condition in my young body, incredibly debilitating bouts of hives, joint problems that ultimately necessitated surgery in both knees, and a weakened nervous system. As is typical in our country I had been raised on meat from a very early age. As a natural vegetarian (although I didn't find this out until the age of 31), my inability to digest meat resulted in persistent and painful digestive difficulties. I had a gourmet background (my mother was a talented hostess and an accomplished gourmet cook) and had traveled considerably from early childhood. I was exposed to international cuisine at an early age. As a college student I had the opportunity to work with a French

[2] Robert S. Mendelsohn, M.D. *How to Raise a Healthy Child in Spite of Your Doctor.* Chicago: Contemporary Books, Inc., 1984: 46–47. (Italics are Dr Mendelsohn's.)

provincial cook, Armand Ducellier, in Avignon, France. All of this was very much part of my identity and my life-style, and at first it was hard for me to see it as the root of my health problems. But the plain fact was that the foods I had been eating were wreaking havoc on my body, leaving me with no energy to cope with anything else in my life.

When I put into practice the principles that Harvey recommended, which are the same that he has just outlined for you, *I lost 20 pounds! In a matter of only 6 weeks, and for the first time in my adult life, I was proud of and comfortable with the shape of my body.* That is an exhilarating feeling that *everyone* deserves! Even more important for me, however, was my change in outlook. The cloud of depression under which I had been living for years began to lift. I began to experience *whole days* of tranquillity. Only someone who has suffered the drain of mental and physical depression can understand what a breakthrough that can be. As my body worked to put itself back into balance, I could see that I was going to be able to live the productive and fulfilling life that had once been my dream. I felt as if I were coming back to the land of the living!

One thing was apparent from the outset: It would be necessary to shed my traditional gourmet approach to food preparation if I was determined to feel consistently well. This became apparent for me during detoxification[3] as my taste buds would periodically yearn for past addictions, and the indulging of those addictions would immediately make me feel unwell again. Working with Harvey, I began to focus on what people would do when they, like me, became aware of the importance of *healthy* weight loss. How would they

[3] Remember, a most important aspect of detoxification is *healthy weight loss!*

make a comfortable transition from their traditional eating habits? What I needed and what others would need was an exciting new approach to delicious yet nutritious food that would please palates, fulfill physiological needs, *and* permit detoxification. Using my creative energies (which were always at their fullest in the kitchen), and pulling from my extensive background in gourmet cooking and the culinary arts, I began to develop a HIGH-ENERGY approach to *nutritious home cooking* that would satisfy desires for variety and flavor and keep me on a detoxification program, feeling better and stronger with each passing day. Subsequently, in addition to my exposure to and studies of French and Italian haute cuisine and American and ethnic cuisine, I studied food artistry, Chinese food preparation, and the cuisines of India and the Middle East. During that time I also received a masters degree in nutritional science from the American College of Health Science.

Harvey had been involved in Natural Hygiene for 6 years before meeting me, and he was much more comfortable on a regimen of fruits and vegetables than I was. He had already been through the transition period when one gives up many of the foods that are not beneficial and learns to substitute new foods that are. He had aleady conquered most of the cravings that I was just beginning to deal with. Harvey taught me many of the meals that he had enjoyed at the beginning of his transition, but we both realized that for the 'detoxification and permanent slenderizing of America' a very wide variety of meals would have to be developed so that the experience could be enjoyable rather than clinical. Our meals became a real challenge for me to see what I could come up with that would be delicious and satisfying, that the kids would love, and that would be good for *all* of us. It required me to be newly creative with vegetables! Frequently mealtime became a bustling family endeavor. That time was a great deal of fun, and we have wanted our program to maintain that joyous spirit so that one's becoming 'fit for life' can be the wonderful beginning of the *best part of one's life.* These endeavors are the basis of the program that we are presenting to you. These are menus that allow eating to be a celebration for your taste buds and a boon for your body!

They are designed to help you adopt a new eating lifestyle so that you will never again have to deal with the problem of excess weight. They are designed to put you in harmony with your natural body cycles. New menu ideas will be presented allowing you to effortlessly adhere to the principles and begin the all-important detoxification of your body. Once initiated, this detoxification will be ongoing and automatic as long as you adhere to the principles to the best of your ability. Weight loss will also be automatic as your body, given the energy to do so, joyously restores itself to its most comfortable weight. If you enjoy these recipes and find them satisfying, you may be interested in referring to my first recipe book, *The Common Sense Guide to a New Way of Eating,*[4] which offers many different ideas for the transition period.

Consider the next 4 weeks a transition period in your life. If you follow the menus outlined, you will automatically be eating fruit correctly, consuming an adequate amount of high-water-content food, and combining your foods properly. In our practice and in the Four-week Detoxification Workshops[5] we have held, we have found that the simplest way to adopt a

[4] Marilyn Diamond. *The Common Sense Guide to a New Way of Eating.* Santa Monica, California: Bantam UK, 1988.

[5] In those four-week workshops, many people *easily* lost between fifteen and twenty-five pounds!

new eating life-style is to follow a step-by-step 4-week *sample* of what that lifestyle would be. Keep in mind that this is precisely what your program is – A SAMPLE. It is not the only regimen that works. That is not what FIT FOR LIFE is all about. What we are giving you here is an *example* of how to use the principles correctly on a daily basis. Our goal is to demonstrate to you the free and creative use of these principles, not to imprison you in a regimen that you use as you have used diets in the past . . . until you got so bored that you had to revert to your old eating habits. That is why you will notice that there are no hard and fast rules in the menu section. Portions are loosely defined. We encourage you to eat to be satisfied and to substitute your favorite ingredients or even a favorite menu item from another day for the examples given. Once you have completed the program, you will know how to eat according to the principles, and you will feel confident about your new eating life-style. If you don't, then repeat it until you do. For some it takes longer than others to learn a new skill. That is what this is – the skill of joyful eating to achieve and maintain your natural body weight.

You now have all the background information that you need. It is time to put the program into practice and experience firsthand . . .

CHAPTER 1

Breakfast

Your morning meals from now on will be a breeze. They will hardly ever vary. **UNTIL NOON EVERY DAY YOU MAY HAVE AS MUCH FRESH FRUIT JUICE AND FRESH FRUIT AS YOU DESIRE.** *This will insure that during the length of the elimination cycle your body will be able to work fully on elimination, not digestion!* Feel free to eat as much fruit as you need to feel satisfied, and, of course, make sure you eat it on an empty stomach. Try to start each day with a fresh fruit juice, if it is available: orange, apple, tangerine, melon, pineapple. Remember that it is most beneficial to make your juice yourself. Make it a top priority to own a juicer – at the very least, a simple citrus juicer.

When desired, have pieces of juicy fruit throughout the morning. *Over a three- to four-hour period we recommend that you have several pieces of fruit.* One serving of fruit is the amount that leaves you feeling comfortable. It may be one orange, or it may be a bowl of four quartered oranges. It may be an apple, or it may be two peaches sliced and sprinkled with a tablespoon of currants. It may be half a cantaloupe or a 3-inch-thick slice of watermelon. It may be a banana or two bananas. Fruit consumption is an art to be developed by each individual. What matters is that you eat enough to feel satisfied. It does not matter if that requires one piece or a large platter full. In Harvey's words, 'Some like to have fruit in the morning, some like to have juice, others prefer warm water with lemon juice. The most important thing I can tell you is that we are not intending to give you some ironclad laws not to be violated or digressed from in any way. Rather, these are principles to be *conveniently* fitted into your personal life-style.'

Learn to listen to the wants and needs of your body. DON'T OVEREAT AND DON'T UNDEREAT! DO BE SATISFIED! Neither stuff yourself to compensate for the emptiness you may feel from missing your customary heavier breakfast nor skip the fruit because you don't feel like having it. YOU NEED THE FRUIT! It supplies the water content and fuel that are so necessary for detoxification.

As the morning progresses, if you feel hungry and are beginning to crave heavier foods, have a couple of bananas. They stay in your stomach a little longer than juicy fruits and give you a fuller feeling. It is fine to have more than one. Be sure that they are ripe, not green. The green indicates that the starch has not yet turned to sugar. Brown spots on the skin of the banana indicate that the starch has been converted to sugar.

Dates and dried fruit should not be eaten at all during the period when you are concentrating on weight loss. Although they are wonderful natural energy foods, they are so full of concentrated sugar that they will inhibit weight loss. Since it is easy to overeat them, it is best to avoid them completely until you have lost at least some of the weight you wish to lose. Ultimately, when you are nearing your ideal weight, you will find them to be a perfect solution to a craving for unwholesome processed sweets. Initially, however, they can be counterproductive, especially if you lack self-control.

An important rule to review is that you may eat fruit of a juicy nature until twenty minutes to one half hour before you eat lunch. Allow about forty-five minutes for banana to pass out of your stomach. Melons have the highest water content of any fruit. It is recommended that they be eaten *before* other fruit, because they pass through the stomach more quickly.

If you like to sit down to a meal in the morning, try a fruit salad. If you have children, try, little by little, to start off their day with fresh juice and a fruit salad too. Even though they may be addicted to overly large, ill-combined breakfasts, if they make the transition to fruit in the morning, they will have much more energy for their work than when their bodies were forced to expend energy on the demands of the digestive tract.

When we first began to develop the program, my two children were both in elementary school. It took over a year to help them break the habit of a large morning meal. I never put pressure on them. I did, however, always make sure that *fruit* was the *first* food in the morning. Then, if they were still not satisfied, I offered a slice of whole-grain toast and raw butter, or granola and apple juice, or even better, I hit on the idea of giving them bowls of piping hot steamed vegetables after their fruit in the morning. At least that way they were still staying on high-water-content food during the all-important elimination cycle. At least bowls of steamed vegetables are *real,* wholesome foods, unlike those multicolored packages of chemically laden imitation foods pushed on our young by the processed food industries.

Once my children were able to make the transition to fruit in the morning, it became clear to them how tired heavier food before noon made them feel. As the years went by they rarely sought anything but fruit before lunch. Their health generally improved, and while other children had frequent colds, they did not. I attributed this to the fact that their elimination cycles were being allowed to function regularly without interruption. Even now, as teenagers, they rarely eat anything before noon but fruit.

With the birth of our son 7 years ago, Harvey and I were able to verify even more clearly the definite advantage of feeding only fruit to children in the morning. Since the elimination cycle, from birth, was rarely interrupted by the consumption of heavy food before noon, he did not develop the mucous nose, the earaches, and the coughs that most young children experience and that their parents come to expect as routine. Our child was never stuffed up or blocked with mucous waste, because his body was allowed *every day* to complete its elimination cycle. His little system was not forced to store waste, unlike those of so many children, whose bodies from morning to night are being forced to deal with an onslaught of heavy food. As an infant and toddler we found him to be happy and even-tempered. At the age of 7 he is tall, well-coordinated, and energetic.

The mothers I have worked with in my practice and in our workshops have seen the same results. Once their children were beginning to be 'weaned' from heavier breakfasts and were, for the most part, consuming fruit or vegetables in the morning and eating foods that were pure rather than laden with chemicals, their overall health began to improve. In one case two young girls at a school for children with learning disabilities in Southern California made such a marked improvement once they had been put on the program that teachers at the school contacted the parents to find out what was bringing about the positive changes.

The key with children is not to apply pressure. (This is also true for some of the childlike adults you may wish to influence!) Pressure causes tension. Where food is concerned, tension is always to be avoided. No matter how good the food might be, if it is eaten under pressure or in a tense environment, it will most often spoil in an agitated digestive tract. Initially, simply make a fruit salad alternative available to your child. Eat it with your child with an air of celebration, so the positive experience is shared. This is fun! Offer bowls of buttery steamed vegetables as alternatives to children's junky cereals. Offer buttered whole-grain toast. At least your children will be eating *real* food. Little by little the transition will be made. Set the example by eating fruit in the morning yourself, and ultimately the kids will follow.

BREAKFAST GUIDELINES

1. Start your day with **FRESH** fruit juice if you desire. Recommended quantity: eight to fourteen ounces.
2. Throughout the morning have pieces of fruit as you feel hungry.
3. Have a *minimum* of 2 servings of fruit in any 3-hour period.
4. Your maximum fruit intake should be governed by your needs. Have as much as you desire. Do not undereat or overeat fruit!
5. Eat melons before other fruit.
6. Eat bananas when you are particularly hungry and are craving heavier food.

CHAPTER 2

Fresh Juices

You will notice as you proceed on the program that juices play a very important part. FRESH JUICES! The kind you make yourself with your own juicer or are made for you at a juice bar. Also available are fresh juices bottled daily by local juice companies. Consider owning your own juicer. This is the most economical way to go, since every time you buy juice, you are paying for someone else's juicer.

In this era of great preoccupation over food supplements, with millions of people regularly consuming expensive pills in the name of nutrition, fresh juices are actually the finest, most real form of supplementation, although most people are totally unaware of it. *All the nutrients that the human body requires are present in balanced quantities in fresh fruits and vegetables. And they can be used by our bodies only when they are consumed as part of the whole food in which they occur.* So it is actually true that a diet rich in fresh fruit and vegetables and their juices supplies *all* the nutritional needs of the body. Juices are the next best thing to the whole food, being merely a liquid extract of the whole food. They are not overly concentrated, as are megavitamin doses, nor have they been processed or 'pharmaceuticalized' in any way. When they are made, you can see what they come from. There is very little difference between the real thing (whole fruits and vegetables) and their juices. They supply us with the vital building blocks for cell regeneration, and in this way they are a true longevity food. (You might want to check the latest books by Dr Norman W. Walker, the fruit and vegetable juice proponent in Arizona who is 109 years old, if you have any questions about juices and longevity!)

There's an added benefit from juices: Their delicious flavors quench our thirst and satisfy us so that we tend less and less to reach for the harmful thirst-quenchers like sodas, coffee, tea, milk, and alcohol. Other than mother's milk, there is no finer food for infants and young children than juice.

We strongly encourage you to get into the habit of consuming fresh juices. They are the *only* beverage that supplies **REAL, VITAL ENERGY**, notwithstanding the false claims made in advertising for other, harmful beverages. The habit of drinking diet sodas just because millions of dollars in advertising have been spent to convince you that they are a 'weight-loss food' is the result of an unscrupulous advertising campaign *against* your well-being. A mixture of laboratory chemicals can only *add* toxins to your body, not help remove them. Diet sodas do nothing but undermine your health and vitality! If you are interested in knowing about other foods that are touted as beneficial but are actually harmful, consult Harvey's first book, *A Case for Health.*[1]

Juices that are fresh are the only beverages that can help you lose weight and feel great. **DRINK THEM ON AN**

[1] Harvey Diamond. *A Case for Health.* Santa Monica, California: Golden Glow Publishers, 1979.

EMPTY STOMACH, NOT WITH OR IMMEDIATELY FOLLOWING ANY OTHER FOOD! Enjoy them! They are extremely beneficial. Remember to drink them slowly, mixing them with your saliva. Gulped or consumed too rapidly, they may upset the blood sugar level.

Considering the importance of fresh juices, owning your own juicer makes a lot of sense. There are many on the market, but we have room here to name only a few. The Champion is an excellent *all-around* juicer, since it is easy to use and clean, makes high-quality juice, and can be used to make nut butters and delicious nondairy frozen desserts. The Ultra-Matic is exclusively for juice extraction, but it is a high-quality precision instrument. It is more expensive than the Champion but well worth the money. The Oster is a sturdy, reasonably priced juicer of great versatility. Oster and Panasonic also make sturdy, inexpensive citrus juicers. For more information on these and other juicers, you can contact the authors by writing to Golden Glow, 2210 Wilshire Blvd., Suite 118, Santa Monica, CA 90403.

CHAPTER 3

The Energy Ladder

A.M.
FRESH FRUIT & FRUIT JUICES
FRESH VEGETABLE JUICES & SALADS
STEAMED VEGETABLES, RAW NUTS, & SEEDS
GRAINS, BREADS, POTATOES, LEGUMES
MEAT, CHICKEN, FISH, DAIRY
P.M.

We have designed the Energy Ladder to help you be more productive and effective during the day while at the same time allowing your body to work at the elimination of toxic waste. It indicates which foods to eat early in the day (fruits and vegetables) and which to eat later when you have accomplished your work for the day and can rest and allow your body to focus its remaining energy on digestion – potatoes, grains, dairy products, and flesh foods. Of course, the foods closest to 'A.M.' can be eaten anytime of the day, but those closest to 'P.M.' should not be eaten early in the day, when you need your energy for so much else. (If an individual's schedule is different from the norm – working at night, sleeping during the day – with total consistency, the body cycles will adjust to that schedule. There is little documentation on this subject, but based on our own observations, this is true.) Any day on which fruits and vegetables are all you consume and meat, grains, or dairy are not eaten at all will be a high-energy, maximum weight-loss day! The menus of the program are based on the Energy Ladder.

CHAPTER 4

The FIT FOR LIFE Shopping List

When people begin to make changes in their eating life-style, they are sometimes surprised (pleasantly) by the variety of foods they are 'still permitted to eat.' We have so frequently heard 'You mean, I can have *this*?' that we have decided to include a shopping list. It is designed to indicate what is available to you so that you will fully understand how unrestrictive we intend this program to be. It also includes some recommended brands that we have found to complement the spirit of this approach. Although all the items may not be available in your supermarket or natural food store, they have been included so you will know what to request. I have intentionally listed items from substantial companies which will be able to increase their distribution as demand increases.

Because of space limitations, I have not been able to list *all* of the many companies that are consciously working to make excellent additive-free products. It is up to you, and I strongly encourage you, to *read labels* and *avoid any* products containing chemicals. Brands you may find that are not mentioned here and that are chemical-free are certainly worth substituting for the ones that do contain chemicals. *Remember, chemicals in your food are toxins in your body!* Many of the items listed were at one time only available in natural food stores and are now more and more accessible in supermarkets. It is greatly to our benefit to have pure, chemical-free products in our supermarkets – so be sure to request them!

It is imperative for you to realize that *this is not a shopping list of required foods.* We would *not* want you to run out and spend a week's pay and a whole weekend trying to fit all that is on this list into your refrigerator and pantry! The list will merely help you become aware of the wide scope of foods that are available to play a role in the changes you make. If your needs can be totally satisfied by only a few of the items listed, that's fine! If not, use this list as a guide to the enormous number of choices that are open to you.

FRUIT

Many fruits used to be available only in certain seasons. Now widespread importing brings us year-round many varieties that used to be seasonal. Importing also allows us to benefit from diverse nutrients from a variety of soils and from a wide range of farming techniques. Some of the many varieties are indicated under each fruit to encourage you to take advantage of the cornucopia of possibilities. A short description of some of the more exotic fruits is also provided.

If you are an 'apples-oranges-bananas person' and that satisfies you, then stay with what you like. If, on the other hand, you feel like experimenting, this list will give you some great ideas. Remember that fruit must *never be cooked,* since cooking transforms its alkalinity to acid.

Many varieties will be listed, but not *all,* because there are so very many. If you come across a certain variety that is not listed, just add it to your list and try it. The beautiful thing about fruit is that **ALL FRUIT IS GOOD NO MATTER WHAT THE VARIETY**, and we are the fortunate benefactors of all this fantastic diversity.

APPLES

Golden Delicious
Granny Smith (green)
Pink Lady
McIntosh
New Zealand Gala (yellow)
Pippin (green, also called Newton)
Red Delicious

APRICOTS

BANANAS

apple bananas (Both apple bananas and red bananas must be *very* ripe before eating, or the consistency will be starchy.)
red
yellow (ripe when spotted)

BERRIES

blackberries
boysenberries
raspberries
blueberries
mulberries
strawberries

CHERRIES

Bing
Royal Anne (a yellow-orange variety)

DATES

Barhi
Deglet Noor (flavor of caramel, chewy)
Medjool (largest, 'the king of the dates')
honey
Khadrawi (soft and almost skinless)

FIGS

Black Mission
Kadota
Calimyrna

GRAPEFRUIT

pink (usually the sweetest)
white

GRAPES

Concord
Muscat of Alexandria
Ribier
Emperor
Red Flame Seedless
Thompson Seedless

MELONS

cantaloupe
Crenshaw
orange flesh honeydew
pink honeydew
watermelon
casaba
honeydew
Persian
Sharlyn

NECTARINES

ORANGES

blood
navel
Valencia

PEACHES

Babcock (white flesh, sweet)
freestone
Suncrest
clingstone
Elberta
Indian Red

PEARS

Anjou
Bartlett
Bosc
Comice
red
Winter Nellis

PINEAPPLES

Hawaiian
Mexican

PLUMS

elephant
greengage
prunes
Red Beaut
Santa Rosa

TANGELOS

(very juicy, slightly tart)

TANGERINES

Keno
mandarin oranges
Satsuma

EXOTIC FRUITS

Many exotic fruits and vegetables have recently been introduced to the American market by Frieda of California. Based in Los Angeles, Frieda's products are sold nationwide. She sells to *every retailer* in the United States and is dedicated to the expansion of the produce market in this country. Frieda is *not* set up to sell mail-order, nor does she sell to the individual consumer. To get her exotic products, request them at your supermarket.

CHERIMOYA

Commonly referred to as 'the aristocrat of fruits,' this heart-shaped fruit has a skin that looks like an alligator's but inside is a puddinglike treat unlike any other you have ever tasted. Slice into wedges and eat off the skin, or cut in half and eat with a spoon. Available in winter through spring.

GUAVA
Shiny green-skinned fruit, small and oblong, these can be cut in half and the sweet green and purple pulp scooped out with a spoon. They are slightly soft when ripe. Available in winter and spring.

KIWI
Fuzzy, brown-skinned fruit, usually the size of a lemon; tangy, bright lime-green inside with tiny edible black seeds. Peel and eat whole, or slice, or cut in half and eat with a spoon. Ripe when soft like a peach.

LOQUAT
Small, pale orange fruit, shiny skin, these grow in clusters on a branch. They turn from green to yellow or orange when ripe. Can be peeled or not. Delicate, juicy orange flesh, large brown seed. Throw the seeds into your garden. They sprout easily into trees in tropical or semitropical climates.

LYCHEE
Small, nutlike, hard brown or reddish skin. Peel to discover pearl-white, juicy pulp with brown seed in center. Rare in United States. Available for a short time during summer. Although difficult to find fresh (they are usually canned), they have a refreshing flavor that, once tasted, is never forgotten.

MANGO
Many varieties, from large (grapefruit-size) red Haydens to oblong yellow-green Haitians. Thick skin should be peeled to reveal deep orange flesh. Can be sliced or eaten whole. Large seed in center, to which

the rich and aromatic fruit clings. Available in late spring and summer.

PAPAYA

Greenish, yellow-orange skin, round or oblong fruit. Hawaiian papayas are the size of an average hand. Mexican papayas can be as large as a small watermelon, but they have a thin, gamey flavor which is less attractive than the sweeter, richer Hawaiian variety. Flesh may be bright orange or strawberry-colored. Ripe when skin turns yellow-orange and fruit gives to pressure. Black seeds at center are bitter and should *not* be eaten. Available year-round.

PERSIMMON

Many varieties, from yellow-orange flat-round Fuyus to deep red-orange soft oval Hychias. Both are close to apples in size, and Fuyus are eaten crisp like apples. Hychias must be *very* soft before they are ripe. The thin skin can be peeled or not. Thick orange custardlike flesh with few or no seeds. Available in the fall.

POMEGRANATE

Pinkish red-skinned fruit. Hard to the touch, about the size of a softball. Cut when hard into quarters to reveal crimson fruit, bittersweet in flavor. Fruit is made up of tiny juicy segments, each one containing a seed. Children love to suck the fruit off the seeds and spit out the seeds. Adults rarely have that much time! Available in the fall.

SAPOTE

Round, green-skinned fruit, white custardlike flesh. Only ripe when *very* soft. Very rare. Available in the winter.

VEGETABLE FRUITS

These are frequently regarded as vegetables but are actually classified botanically as fruits, because they contain seeds. Vegetable fruits combine raw with other fruits: for example, avocado with banana, papaya, or mango; cucumber with peaches, oranges, or nectarines. They also combine well with all raw or cooked vegetables and with starchy carbohydrates such as bread, rice, pasta, or potatoes. Ideally, vegetable fruits should *never* be cooked, although we will once in a while make an exception for peppers. You would *never* cook avocado, cucumber, and particularly tomato. Tomatoes become *very* acid when cooked and acidify your whole system. Eat vegetable fruits *raw,* as an alternative to sweet fruits when you want something *juicy* but not sweet.

Except for avocado, which stays in the stomach for an hour at most, all the juicy vegetable fruits can be combined with other fruits with no extra waiting time.

AVOCADO

Bacon
Haas
Topa-Topa
Fuerte
Pinkerton

CUCUMBER

hothouse
standard
pickling cukes

PEPPERS

bell – green or red
green chili

TOMATOES

(Tomatoes are exceedingly acid-forming when cooked, so eat them uncooked. Raw, they are extremely alkaline and beneficial.)

DRIED FRUITS

These are extremely concentrated and should be eaten in small quantities. Dried fruit can be eaten sparingly with other, less sweet fruits to augment their sweetness. Avoid all fruit that has been sulfur-dried. Only sun-dried fruit is recommended.

APPLES	**APRICOTS**	**BANANAS**
CURRANTS	**FIGS**	**MANGO**
PAPAYA	**PEACHES**	**PEARS**
PINEAPPLES	**PRUNES**	**RAISINS**

(Thompson Seedless, monukka)

VEGETABLES

Buy these *fresh* when you can. Buy frozen when fresh are not available.

ARTICHOKES

ASPARAGUS

BEETS

BOK CHOY (Similar to Swiss chard, but saltier.)

BROCCOLI

BRUSSELS SPROUTS

CABBAGE Napa (Chinese), new (white), red, savoy

CARROTS

CAULIFLOWER

CELERY

CELERY ROOT (Celeriac)

CHARD green, red

CORN

DAIKON (Japanese radish)

DANDELION GREENS

EGGPLANT

BELGIAN ENDIVE

FENNEL
(The root can be braised or sliced raw into salads. The leaf and seed are used as herbs.)

GARLIC

GREEN BEANS (string beans)

JERUSALEM ARTICHOKE (sunchoke)

JICAMA (tropical tuber)

KALE

LEEKS

LETTUCE

arugula	Boston or Bibb (butter)
chicory	escarole
iceberg	limestone
radicchio	romaine
salad bowl	

LIMA BEANS

MUSHROOMS
(fresh, or dried if fresh are not available)
cepes (porcini) (Available by mail from Todaro Bros., 557 Second Ave., New York, NY 10016 [212] 679-7766)
chanterelles (Available by mail from H. Roth and Son, 1577 First Ave., New York, NY 10028, [212] 734-1111)

common cultivated
enoki
morels
oyster
shiitake
straw (The Asian mushrooms are available fresh and dried in Asian markets and many supermarkets.)
wood ear

MUSTARD GREENS

ONIONS

Bermuda (red)
white
spring or scallions
yellow

PARSNIPS

PEAS

POTATOES

new (red-skinned)
sweet potatoes
yams
Yellow Finnish (A new variety distributed by Frieda of California, these look like a small russet but have a yellow, *very* creamy pulp.)
Russet Burbank
White Rose

RADISHES

RUTABAGAS

SEA VEGETABLES

(The best brands are from Westbrae Natural Foods, 4240 Hollis St., Emeryville, CA 94608, and Eden Foods, 701 Tecumseh Rd., Clinton, MI 49236.)

arame
hiziki
nori
dulse
kombu
wakame

SHALLOTS

SNAP BEANS (edible pods)

SNOW PEAS (sugar peas)

SPINACH

SPROUTS

aduki
alfalfa
buckwheat
fenugreek
lentil
mung bean
pea
radish
red clover
red lentil
sunflower

SQUASH (Summer)

crookneck (yellow)
pattipan (summer)
scallopini
zucchini

SQUASH (Winter)

acorn
banana
butternut
Chinese
delicata
golden acorn
hubbard
Japanese
pumpkin
sweet dumpling
turban
Turkish

TURNIPS

WATERCRESS

WAX BEANS

NUTS

All nuts should be eaten raw. In this state they are *highly concentrated* in nutrition and completely usable in the human system. As a source of protein (high-quality amino acids) and calcium, they leave no toxic residue in the body as do dairy and flesh sources. Remember, however, that nuts as a protein source are more difficult to break down than fruits and vegetables, and they are extremely concentrated. *Avoid overeating nuts, and never eat them roasted.* Roasted nuts are terribly acidifying to the system. Raw nuts are an excellent source of natural oil. NOTE: When eating nuts at a meal, do not eat any other concentrated food.

ALMONDS

BRAZIL NUTS

CASHEWS

COCONUTS (fresh or dried, *never* sweetened)

FILBERTS

MACADAMIA NUTS

PECANS

PIGNOLIAS (pine nuts)

PISTACHIOS

WALNUTS

SEEDS

Like nuts, seeds are a concentrated source of protein that should be eaten raw, never roasted, and in small quantities. Never combine seeds with any other concentrated food.

CARAWAY

POPPY

PUMPKIN

SESAME

SUNFLOWER

SEED AND NUT BUTTERS

These are always preferable raw rather than roasted. Roasted, they will have an acidifying effect. For best digestion, combine nut butters with raw vegetables. Whipped with water, they make a great dip. Peanuts are not actually nuts, but legumes. Peanut butter is harder to digest than nut and seed butters. (Hain products can be ordered from Hain Pure Food Company, 13660 S. Figueroa, Los Angeles, CA 90061.)

ALMOND (Hain unsalted raw)

CASHEW (Westbrae)

SESAME (tahini – Westbrae)

SUNFLOWER (Hain unsalted raw)

GRAINS

BREADS (whole-grain or sprouted)

Food for Life brand flourless breads
- Ezekiel 4:9
- Sprouted 7 Grains
- whole-wheat

Food for Life brand bran muffins, carrot muffins, sprouted wheat burger buns

Food for Life wheat-free rice bread

Garden of Eatin' Sproutbreads – sliced
- ONEderful
- seeded rye
- Sproutcake
- Too Many Raisins Bread

Lifestream brand Essene Bread

Oasis flourless breads

sprouted corn
sprouted rye
sprouted wheat

chapatis (Cedarlane, Garden of Eatin')
corn tortillas (Cedarlane, Natural and Kosher)
pita bread (whole-wheat)
Thin-Thin bread – Garden of Eatin'
Whole Wheat Tortillas – Garden of Eatin'

BARLEY

COUSCOUS (Couscous is considered a grain, although it is actually a tiny pasta made from semolina, flour, water, and salt. It is precooked, dried, and then rehydrated when used. There are many ways to serve it, but the word *couscous* only *really* connotes the grain.)

CRACKED WHEAT (bulgur)

KASHA (buckwheat groats)

MILLET

RICE

basmati
brown
sweet
wild

CEREALS

Familia
granola (honey-sweetened or unsweetened – Eden)

CHIPS

We recommend eating a good quality low-salt or salt-free chip with vegetables or salad – if you are craving chips.

Ananda's Salt-Free Chips
Barbara's (unsalted)
Dr Bronner's Corn & Sesame Snack Chips

Eden chips
Edward & Sons Brown Rice Wheels and vegetable chips
Hav-A-Corn-Chips
Health Valley (unsalted)
Kettle Chips (unsalted)
Mother Earth tortilla chips
Soken – Seaweed Crunch, mushroom, carrot, vegetable, and Vege Soy

CRACKERS (any whole-grain variety without chemical additives, sugar, cheese, or preservatives)

Ak-mak
Finn Crisp
Health Valley
Mi-Del Honey Grahams
rice cakes (Arden and Chico-San)
Wasa Crisp Bread
Westbrae Unsalted Brown Rice Wafers

PASTAS
artichoke
corn
ramen and soba (Westbrae, Eden, Soken)
sesame
Vegeroni
vegetable
whole-wheat (De Cecco, Westbrae, Eden)

FLOUR AND MEAL
cornmeal (El Molino)
  yellow
  white
graham flour
rye flour (El Molino, Arrowhead Mills)
whole-wheat flour (El Molino, Arrowhead Mills)
whole-wheat pastry flour (El Molino)

If you cannot find some of these products in your natural food store or supermarket, ask your retailer to contact these excellent sources, or write to them yourself:

Food for Life, 3580 Pasadena Avenue, Los Angeles, CA 90031
Lifestream Natural Foods, Ltd., 12411 Vulcan Way, Richmond, B.C., Canada V6V 137
Oasis Health Breads, Inc., P.O. Box 182, 440 Venture St., Escondido, CA 92025
Cedarlane, 4928 Hollywood Blvd., Hollywood, CA 90027
Natural and Kosher Foods, Inc., Los Angeles, CA 90061
Garden of Eatin', 5300 Santa Monica Blvd., Hollywood, CA 90029
Soken Trading, Inc., 591 Redwood Hwy., Suite 2125, Mill Valley, CA 94941
El Molino Mills, 345 N. Baldwin Park Blvd., City of Industry, CA 91746
Arrowhead Mills, Inc., Hereford, TX 79045
Sovex Natural Foods, Box 310, Collegedale, TN 37315
Health Valley Natural Foods, Montebello, CA 90640
Ak Mak-Ararat Bakeries, Div. of Soojian, Inc., 89 Academy Ave., Sanger, CA 93657
Finn Crisp – Wasa Bread – Shaffer-Clarke, Inc., Old Greenwich, CT 06870
Mi-Del Honey Grahams – Health Foods, Inc., Des Moines, IA 60018
Rice Cakes – Arden Organics, Inc., 99 Pond Rd., Asheville, NC 28806
Ananda Products – 918 N. Broadway, Box 24125, Oklahoma City, OK 73124
Barbara's Chips – Barbara's Bakery, Inc., Novato, CA 94947

Dr Bronner's All-One-God-Faith, Inc., Box 28, Escondido, CA 92025

Edward and Sons, Union, NJ 07083

Hav-A-Corn – Hav-A Natural Foods, Box 964, Laguna Beach, CA 92651

Kettle Chips – N.S. Khalsa, Box 664, Salem, OR 97308

Mother Earth Chips – Enterprises, Inc., U.S. Naturals Corp., Novato, CA 94947

LEGUMES

ADUKI BEANS

BLACK-EYED PEAS (cowpeas)

GARBANZO BEANS (chickpeas)

GREAT NORTHERN BEANS

KIDNEY BEANS

LENTILS (red and brown)

LIMA BEANS

MUNG BEANS

NAVY BEANS

PINTO BEANS

SPLIT PEAS (yellow and green)

DAIRY PRODUCTS

All dairy products should be unpasteurized (raw) *whenever possible.* Although there are medical concerns pertaining to raw vs. unpasteurized dairy products, the controversy may be more commercial than scientific in nature. Notwithstanding the unresolved debate that currently exists, numerous individuals find their health and well-being immeasurably enhanced through the avoidance of unnecessarily pasteurized products. (Alta Dena Dairies, City of Industry, CA 91747, has a full line of delicious, high-quality raw dairy products.)

BUTTER (unsalted)

SOUR CREAM

WHIPPING CREAM

WHITE CHEESES (Yellow cheeses are dyed.)

YOGURT (plain, cow's or goat's milk)

MEAT AND FISH

Since saturated fats are always to be avoided, pork is the *least* desirable meat, beef is the second least desirable, and duck is third. *Any* cured or salted meats or fish are not recommended (frankfurters, sausages, smoked fish). Buy naturally grazed meat and poultry when it is available. Shelton Farms Poultry, Pomona, CA 91767, is naturally corn-fed and available in many natural food stores. (Beware of parasites – avoid eating your meat or fish raw!) Buy fresh or frozen fish, rather than canned, whenever possible.

CHICKEN

CORNISH HENS

FISH

SEAFOOD

TURKEY

OILS

Should be unrefined and cold-pressed, if possible.

ALMOND (Hain)

AVOCADO (Hain)

CORN (Arrowhead Mills, Eden)

OLIVE (Golden Eagle, Old Monk, Williams-Sonoma [mail order], Westbrae), or any cold-pressed or first-pressing olive oil you prefer. There are scores available at a wide range of prices. 'Extra Virgin' is the finest grade and is almost always cold-pressed.

PEANUT (Arrowhead Mills)

SAFFLOWER (Arrowhead Mills, Eden, Hain, Hollywood, Westbrae; Hollywood safflower oil is distributed more widely than any of the others. I have found Hollywood to be comparable to Hain oil. They are made by Hain-Hollywood, and Hollywood is more widely distributed and *lower* in price. Hollywood Oil: Hollywood Health Foods, Los Angeles, CA 90061.)

SESAME (Eden, Hain, Westbrae)

SALAD DRESSINGS

Any that are pure, containing no sugar, vinegar, or chemicals: Aware Inn, Cardini's, Hain, Health Valley, The Source. (Cesar Cardini Foods, Culver City, CA 90230.)

SEASONINGS AND CONDIMENTS

BARBECUE SAUCE
Hain
Robbie's (Robbie's Natural Products, 3191 Grandeur Ave., Altadena, CA 91001)

KUZU or **ARROWROOT** (Westbrae)

MAYONNAISE (any without sugar – Hain Saf-flower, Hollywood [Rich in Safflower], Westbrae)

MISO (Cold Mountain, Eden, Westbrae)

MUSTARD
Albert Lucas' 100% Natural Mustard (no salt) (Albert Lucas, 25 Rue Royale, 75008 Paris, France)
Grey Poupon
Gulden's Spicy Brown
Hain unsalted

OLIVES (any without acid preservatives or vinegar)
Capello's (Capello's Gourmet Food Products, Buena Park, CA 91062)
Graber (C. C. Graber Co., Ontario, CA 91761)

PICKLES (dill – any without preservatives)
Cosmic Cukes (Pure & Simple, Inc., Corona, CA 91720)
Pure & Simple (same)

SALT SUBSTITUTES (should contain no MSG or sugar)
Ananda Low Sodium Seasoning (Ananda Products, 918 W. Broadway, Box 24125, Oklahoma City, OK 73124)
Bragg Liquid Aminos (Live Food Products, Santa Barbara, CA 93102)
Dr Bronner's seasonings – dry and liquid
dulse flakes or powder

Herbit (Presco Food Products, Flemington, NJ 08822)
kelp granules or powder
Parsley Patch salt-free herbal blends (Parsley Patch, Inc., P.O. Box 2043, Santa Rosa, CA 95405)

SEA SALT (Pure & Simple, Westbrae)

SEASONED SALTS (Gayelord Hauser Products, Modern Products, Inc., 3015 W. Vera Ave., Milwaukee, WI 53209)

Onion Magic
Vege-Sal
Spike
Vegit

SOY SAUCE and **TAMARI** (low-sodium – Eden, Soken, Westbrae)

TOFU SAUCE (Westbrae)

VEGETABLE BOUILLON and **BROTH**
Gayelord Hauser
Hügli (K & L, Box 54606, Tulsa, OK 74115)
Morga (Morga Ag, 9652 Ebnat-Kappel/Suisse)
Vegex (Vegex Co., Division of Presco Food Products, Inc., Flemington, NJ 08822)

HERBS

Gayelord Hauser Products (Modern Products, Inc., 3015 W. Vera Ave., Milwaukee, WI 53209) puts up very pure herbs under the Spike brand name. There are many companies offering the herbs listed here, but some put chemical additives in their products.

BASIL

BAY LEAF

CELERY SEED

CHERVIL

CILANTRO

DILL SEED

DILL WEED

FENNEL

KARI LEAVES *(neam)**
MARJORAM
OREGANO
PARSLEY
PEPPERMINT
ROSEMARY
SAGE
SUMMER SAVORY
TARRAGON
THYME

SPICES

Spike brand spices by Gayelord Hauser are the best.

ALLSPICE
ASAFETIDA *(hing)***
CARDAMOM
CAYENNE
CINNAMON
CLOVES
CORIANDER
CUMIN
CURRY
GINGER
MACE
MUSTARD SEEDS***
NUTMEG
PAPRIKA
RED PEPPER
SAFFRON
SWEET HUNGARIAN PAPRIKA
TURMERIC
WHITE PEPPER

*An Indian herb available at Indian markets, not available from Spike.
**An Indian spice available at Indian markets, not from Spike.
***Available at Indian markets, not from Spike.

SWEETENERS

DATE SUGAR

MAPLE SUGAR

MAPLE SYRUP

RAW HONEY *(Legally,* honey can be heated to 160 degrees and *still be termed 'natural.'* But at 130 degrees the honey is made useless due to its resulting acid nature.)

TEAS

Celestial Seasonings, 1780 55th St., Boulder, CO 80301 (We have found this to be an *exceptional* product.)
Seelect Inc., Chatsworth, CA 91311

COFFEE SUBSTITUTES

Cafix (Richter Bros., Inc., Carlstadt, NJ 07072)
Dacopa Foods, California Natural Products, Manteca, CA 95336
Pionier (K & L, Box 54606, Tulsa, OK 74115)
Rombouts, Lawrence Hill Rd. 7, Huntington, NY 11743

CHAPTER 5

The Main-Course Salad

THE HEART OF HIGH-ENERGY WEIGHT LOSS

One of the most exciting and innovative aspects of weight loss and fitness is the main-course salad approach to eating. This is a most convenient tool to have at your fingertips. The people we have worked with directly have easily incorporated this into their eating life-styles and have reaped the many benefits.

The main-course salad is deliciously satisfying, and once you have grasped how easy it is to make, you'll experience how much fun it can be. The basic philosophy behind main-course salad artistry is that with a little ingenuity all the ingredients that go into your meal can become part of one great, high-water-content, properly combined salad. This concept insures that the largest proportion of what you are eating is fresh, live vegetables, and this is its greatest advantage. No matter what you are adding to your salad, the bulk of your meal will still be *live*. Whatever you have added to your salad will break down more quickly and pass through your system more easily due to its properly combined nature and the presence of all the fresh raw vegetables.

Over the years we have developed and perfected at least a score of main-course salads, and we're still coming up with new ones all the time. That's the beauty of this concept – the possibilities are endless! On the following pages you will become acquainted with 7 that we have chosen as the most delectable. These particular 7 salads incorporate a wide range of popular foods, so over the next 4 weeks many of your evening meals will consist of such innovations as Mediterranean Rice Salad (page 247), Curried Chicken Salad (page 258), Award-winning Potato-lovers' Salad (page 271), Steak-lovers' Salad (page 280), California Tostada (page 289), Farmer's Chop Suey (page 307), and Cantonese Seafood Salad (page 330). It's great to sit down to some of your favorite foods as the basis for a completely original salad meal. Until you've eaten these salads, you haven't fully experienced what salad meals can be.

Another truly marvelous part of main-course salads is that they take very little effort to prepare, yet the results are tremendous, from the standpoint of weight loss and health benefits and for the eating experience. And if that's not enough, main-course salads are consistently inexpensive. You will continually be amazed at how economically you can feed yourself, your family, and your friends using this particular approach. These salads also tend to keep well overnight if there are any leftovers, which is unusual. These are winners!

The main-course salads are a vital part of the next 4 weeks of menus. They are designed to help you lose weight and feel great quickly and comfortably. Take advantage of them and enjoy them. They are easy to make, and what will be most rewarding for you is that you will consistently leave the table with a feeling of complete satisfaction. They are interesting, filling meals that not only taste wonderful but also facilitate the loss of weight. **REMEMBER THAT YOU CAN SUBSTITUTE ANY MAIN-COURSE SALAD FOR ANY DINNER MENU. YOU CAN ALSO SUBSTITUTE ONE MAIN-COURSE SALAD FOR ANOTHER.**

A WORD ABOUT SALAD BARS

Salad bars are a great boon to the health-conscious, weight-conscious diner if they are used to best advantage. Sometimes, however, they include such a diversity of raw and cooked food that it is actually possible to return to one's table with a plate full of *anything* but salad. I have observed people returning to their seats holding plates mounded with shrimp salad, potato salad, chicken salad, macaroni salad, pickled herring, garlic toast, and cheesecake. I have had to restrain myself from asking, 'Where's the salad?' as they joyously dug in, remarking, 'Boy, these salad bars are great!' Salad? What they're having is a smorgasbord with dressing!

Here are some tips on how to get the most from any salad bar and walk away feeling satisfied that you've really had a good, high-water-content, properly combined salad. First, before you take a plate, decide what you are going to combine with what at this particular meal. Survey the entire offering. In handling food combinations at salad bars, it's best to know what's available rather than plunging in without a plan. Some salads or salad items in the layout will be made from concentrated foods; for example, macaroni salad, croutons, and shrimp, crab, or chicken salad. There may be cheeses available as garnishes. If you choose to have a protein such as a meat or cheese, forgo all carbohydrates such as beans, bread, and potato or macaroni salads. If you wish to have beans, potato salad, bread, or a *little* of each, forgo *all* protein. A protein and a carbohydrate consumed simultaneously will not digest properly, and a protein and a protein won't, but more than one carbohydrate, such as beans and croutons, although not ideal, can be consumed at the same time *as long as high-water-content food still predominates the meal.* Whatever concentrated foods you choose to include in the meal, make sure the bulk of your salad still consists of high-water-content vegetables.

By the way, if the salad bar has a fresh fruit salad or a fruit display, and you have time, by all means feel free to have some before your vegetable salad, as long as you have eaten no other food but fruit for three hours and your stomach is empty. Then wait twenty minutes or so for the fruit salad to pass out of your stomach, and you can then begin to prepare your vegetable salad.

We are very often asked, 'What shall I do about the salad dressings at salad bars? Aren't they full of sugar, chemicals, and vinegar?' Unfortunately at many salad bars this is the case; however, it really is not a grave problem. There are plenty of ways around it. Many salad bars have lemon wedges and oil available, so you can have a simple lemon or oil-and-lemon dressing. Many offer a choice of several dressings, at least one of which will be acceptable. I personally know many people who are so dedicated to this life-style that when they go to a salad bar where they are unsure of the dressings, they simply bring their own. On occasion we have stopped at a natural food store on the way to an unfamiliar salad bar to purchase a bottle of dressing without chemical additives or sugar, simply to have it as a backup in case there were no dressings we were interested in using. Several years ago we were working with a group of young, dynamic salesmen who thought nothing of packing a flask of dressing in their attaché cases for their daily stop at the salad bar. Not that you should become fanatical! If the worst thing you ever do dietetically is have a slightly inferior salad dressing on your salad, we'll get together when you're 80 for some tennis! The quality of dressings at salad bars will improve as more and more people begin to demand it.

Salad bars are a timely American innovation. It seems appropriate that the country that has led the world in junk food consumption now has the opportunity to turn that trend toward salad bars – a far more positive direction. They are a great culinary concept, offering the opportunity for so much individual creativity in the eating experience. With their abundant displays of fresh *live* food they reinforce feelings of well-being, beauty, and cleanliness that come automatically from the consumption of predominantly live food meals.

CHAPTER 6

Life-style Guidelines

- Remember that this program is merely an *example* of how to eat according to the principles. You may substitute ingredients you prefer in the recipes or leave out what you don't like. Amounts are not always specified because our recommendation is that you eat as much as you need to feel satisfied. The menus are as pure and ideal as we feel we can make them and still be confident that you will enjoy your transition as much as we enjoyed ours. Achieving all the great results we know you will achieve – while enjoying your food – will insure that you will *not frequently* wish to return to a less healthy life-style!
- Use fresh fruit and vegetables whenever possible. Use frozen (without sugar or sauces) when fresh are not available.
- Recipes in the following section are geared for family consumption and not intended just for those wishing to lose weight. Many are kid-tested.
- **ON ANY GIVEN DAY YOU MAY CHOOSE ONE OF THE MAIN-COURSE SALADS AS A SUBSTITUTE FOR THE SUGGESTED DINNER MENU.**

- You may have fruit, if you are hungry, 3 hours after lunch.
- You may have fruit, if you are hungry, 3 hours after dinner.
- Use dressings, condiments, and seasonings without chemical additives and preservatives, sugar, or MSG. These only *add* toxins to your body. (See the shopping list in Chapter Four for alternatives.)
- Avoid vinegar in salad dressings. It is a ferment that suspends salivary digestion and retards the digestion of starches. Substitute lemon juice for vinegar.
- Avoid the excessive consumption of raw onions and garlic. They pervert the taste buds and cause you to crave heavy foods.
- Freeze any leftover soups. They can be used later in the program.
- Use only whole-grain breads.
- Use raw butter and raw dairy products if they are available.
- Fresh fruit or a fresh fruit salad can be substituted for any lunch.
- When cutting back on dairy products, take advantage of raw nuts as an abundant source of calcium. Raw nuts are particularly useful for women who wish to offset the normal drop in calcium at the onset of the menstrual cycle.
- Feel free to substitute produce that you prefer for what is indicated. Use what is fresh in your region rather than resorting to frozen. The program is flexible to take into consideration availability due to

geographic differences. **AS LONG AS THE PRINCIPLES ARE RESPECTED, IT WILL WORK FOR YOU.**

- You can always go lighter than is indicated at any one meal, but try to refrain from ever going heavier. If you do go lighter consistently, you may speed up your detoxification and risk a little discomfort, so try to stick to what is outlined as much as possible.
- Any dish followed by an asterisk will be a new dish with the recipe provided below the menu.
- Approximate preparation times provided for each recipe include the actual cooking time.

DO NOT OVEREAT. DO NOT OVEREAT. DO NOT OVEREAT.
DO NOT OVEREAT. DO NOT OVEREAT. DO NOT OVEREAT.
DO NOT OVEREAT. DO NOT OVEREAT. DO NOT OVEREAT.
DO NOT OVEREAT. DO NOT OVEREAT. DO NOT OVEREAT.
DO NOT OVEREAT. DO NOT OVEREAT. DO NOT OVEREAT.
DO NOT OVEREAT. DO NOT OVEREAT. DO NOT OVEREAT.
DO NOT OVEREAT. DO NOT OVEREAT. DO NOT OVEREAT.
DO NOT OVEREAT. DO NOT OVEREAT. DO NOT OVEREAT.
DO NOT OVEREAT. DO NOT OVEREAT. DO NOT OVEREAT.
DO NOT OVEREAT. DO NOT OVEREAT. DO NOT OVEREAT.
DO NOT OVEREAT. DO NOT OVEREAT. DO NOT OVEREAT.
DO NOT OVEREAT. DO NOT OVEREAT. DO NOT OVEREAT.
DO NOT OVEREAT. DO NOT OVEREAT. DO NOT OVEREAT.
DO NOT OVEREAT. DO NOT OVEREAT. DO NOT OVEREAT.
DO NOT OVEREAT. DO NOT OVEREAT. DO NOT OVEREAT.
DO NOT OVEREAT. DO NOT OVEREAT. DO NOT OVEREAT.
DO NOT OVEREAT. DO NOT OVEREAT. DO NOT OVEREAT.
DO NOT OVEREAT. DO NOT OVEREAT. DO NOT OVEREAT.
DO NOT OVEREAT. DO NOT OVEREAT. DO NOT OVEREAT.
DO NOT OVEREAT. DO NOT OVEREAT. DO NOT OVEREAT.
DO NOT OVEREAT. DO NOT OVEREAT. DO NOT OVEREAT.
DO NOT OVEREAT. DO NOT OVEREAT. DO NOT OVEREAT.
DO NOT OVEREAT. DO NOT OVEREAT. DO NOT OVEREAT.
DO NOT OVEREAT. DO NOT OVEREAT. DO NOT OVEREAT.
DO NOT OVEREAT. DO NOT OVEREAT. DO NOT OVEREAT.
DO NOT OVEREAT. DO NOT OVEREAT. DO NOT OVEREAT.
DO NOT OVEREAT. DO NOT OVEREAT. DO NOT OVEREAT.
DO NOT OVEREAT. DO NOT OVEREAT. DO NOT OVEREAT.

DO NOT OVEREAT!

EVEN THE FINEST, MOST NUTRITIOUS FOOD AVAILABLE WILL SPOIL IN YOUR SYSTEM IF IT IS OVEREATEN. **PLEASE DO NOT OVEREAT**!

DO NOT OVEREAT!

If you tend to overeat, it is helpful to understand the physiology behind overeating. Putting aside psychological causes for this discussion, there are two main physiological causes for overeating. They are important in that they are sometimes easier to deal with and more correct than the psychological causes. Correcting them frequently makes correcting the psychological causes much easier.

One of the reasons that we frequently overeat is that our bodies are not absorbing nutrients. Nutrients are absorbed through the intestines. If the tiny villi, or filaments, through which nutrients are absorbed are clogged, no matter how much we eat, our bodies are not nourished. These villi can be easily clogged by the waste products of foods that our bodies are unable to metabolize and utilize efficiently. When no nutrients are being absorbed as a result of clogging, the body sets off an alarm that it has not been fed, and even though we have just eaten, we want to eat more.

Another reason for overeating is the consumption of nonnutritious foods such as common junk foods, children's processed cereals, and other highly processed foods. Our bodies set off the alarm once again for more food, because they are literally starving . . . NUTRITIONALLY. There is no better way to malnourish your body than to eat processed foods and junk foods excessively. A malnourished body will cry out for food even though the individual is eating large quantities. If they are large quantities of junk food, the body experiences slow starvation. One might say that the reason over 60 per cent of our population is overweight is that we are overeating as we slowly starve ourselves on American junk food.

This new life-style will help you deal with both

causes of overeating. The large amount of high-water-content food will help cleanse the intestines and unclog the villi so that the body can begin to absorb nutrients. Since only wholesome, fresh foods brimming with nutrients are included in the program, your body will begin to be nourished from the foods it is eating. In short, your body will no longer need to sound the alarm for more food, since it will be regularly receiving food that will cleanse it and nourish it.

If initially you still feel the need to overeat, don't be upset. Stay on the program and allow your body to cleanse itself. Eat juicy raw fruit and raw vegetables when the inclination to overeat surfaces. Raw vegetables will be particularly helpful. As you continue to eat these foods that are brimming with nutrients, the physiological basis for overeating will be removed. Eventually, like so many others, you will be able to say, 'I used to overeat.'

A Four-week Example of the Fitness Life-style

DAY ONE – MONDAY

BREAKFAST:

Always the same: fresh-squeezed juice, as much as desired, up to 14 ounces; fresh juicy fruit in a satisfying quantity, *or* a fruit salad; bananas when you are particularly hungry.

If it is convenient, it is sometimes most comfortable to stagger one's fruit intake throughout the morning.

LUNCH:

Fresh fruit juice, *or* fresh carrot juice, 4-8 ounces, if desired.
Energy Salad* with any raw vegetable additions you prefer
and Light Dressing,*
or The Properly Combined Sandwich*
with cucumber or celery spears

DINNER:

Fresh Vegetable Juice Cocktail*
Perfect Creamy Cauliflower Soup*
Potato Boats,* *or* Easy Roast Chicken*
Garlic String Beans*
French Green Salad*

ENERGY SALAD

Serves 1–2. *15 Min.*

- 3 cups lettuce – iceberg, butter, romaine, red leaf, or salad bowl (*or* any combination of these), washed, dried, and broken into bite-size pieces
- 1 cup spinach, coarsely chopped (optional)
- 1 small cucumber *or* 2 pickling cukes, peeled and sliced
- 1 medium tomato, cubed or sliced
- 1–2 cups sprouts – alfalfa, red clover, mung bean, lentil, sunflower, *or* buckwheat (or any combination of these)
- Any raw vegetable additions such as carrots, celery, mushrooms, red *or* green cabbage, jicama, radishes, beets, zucchini, cauliflower, broccoli, *or* Jerusalem artichokes (optional)
- ¼ cup olives *or* several slices avocado (optional)
- ½ cup beans *or* ¼ cup raw sunflower or sesame seeds (optional)

In large bowl, combine all ingredients. Add ¼–⅓ cup Light Dressing (see page 239) *or* dressing of your choice. Toss well. You can be as flexible as you like with this salad and vary the amounts of each ingredient according to your preference. The tomato and cucumber are important and useful, because their extra water content will help in digestion of the more fibrous greens.

LIGHT DRESSING:

Enough for 1 large or *2 small salads.* *5 Min.*

- 1 clove garlic, halved
- 3 tablespoons olive, safflower, *or* unrefined sunflower oil
- 1 tablespoon fresh lemon juice
- ¼ teaspoon sea salt, seasoned salt, *or* salt-free seasoning containing no MSG or other chemicals
- Fresh ground black pepper (optional)

Place all ingredients in measuring cup, and allow to sit for 15 minutes or longer so garlic flavors oil. Pierce garlic with fork, and whip ingredients together with garlic fork. Discard garlic. Pour dressing over salad, and toss well.

THE PROPERLY COMBINED SANDWICH

Serves 1. *5 Min.*

The very nature of the typical sandwich is that it combines a protein and a carbohydrate, and therefore it wastes a great deal of digestive energy. Properly combined sandwiches on whole-grain bread, using tomato, avocado, and cucumber, with lettuce or sprouts as fillings, are delicious and energizing. Always toast your bread lightly to break down the glutens and make it more digestible. Use whatever condiments you desire so that you will really enjoy your sandwich. If you are using tomato and are not going to eat the sandwich immediately, place layers of lettuce or sprouts between the tomato and the bread so the bread will not become soggy.

Let's take a minute here to have a better understanding of the avocado. Avoid *depriving yourself of this unique and delicious food. Its reputation as 'fattening' is unfounded, since it is a natural fat that the human body is biologically adapted to digest with great ease, as long as it is properly combined. Avocado, a vegetable fruit, combines well with starches, such as bread or chips, with all cooked or raw vegetables, and with fruit such as papaya, mango, banana, and orange. Blended with these fruits it makes a terrific natural baby food. I have even seen avocado used on baked potato instead of sour cream and butter.*

Avocado is ripe when the fruit yields slightly to pressure from the thumb. If the avocado is too soft, its oil will be rancid, so avoid buying soft, mushy ones at reduced prices, thinking they will make great guacamole. To work with an avocado most effectively, simply cut the fruit in half the long way. Remove the seed and scoop out the flesh with a spoon. Or you can slice the seeded avocado and peel each slice separately. If you are mashing the avocado but not using it immediately, return the seed to the bowl or add some lemon juice (to keep the mixture from discoloring), cover tightly, and refrigerate. Cut avocado must be wrapped tightly with the seed to store so it will not discolor.

Avocado is such an exquisite food. Once people find that they can *have it, they sometimes go overboard, eating many avocados a day. We recommend* no more than *one half to one large avocado per person on any given day, because until you are accustomed to avocado in your diet, you may too easily overeat it. Another important point about avocados is this: Even though they are a vegetable fruit, they should* not *be combined with a protein, because they inhibit digestion of proteins. Remember, they may be combined with a starch, such as chips (with guacamole) or bread (for an avocado sandwich).* Please note that whatever concerns you may have associating avocado eating with increased cholesterol in the body are *totally unfounded.* The cholesterol you should be concerned about, and rightfully so, is to be found *only* in animal products, *never* in the plant kingdom. This is a time when many prestigious health organizations such as the National Institutes of Health and the American Heart Association are adamantly stressing the extreme importance of lowering cholesterol in one's diet to reduce heart disease. That is precisely what the FIT FOR LIFE eating plan succeeds in accomplishing. With the *help* of avocados!

2	slices whole-grain bread, lightly toasted
2 or 3	thick slices tomato
3 or 4	lengthwise slices cucumber
	Several slices avocado
	Lettuce *or* sprouts
	Mayonnaise, mustard, *or* butter

In making your sandwich, use bread, condiments, and several thick slices of avocado, tomato, and cucumber, *alone or in any combination.* Top with generous handful of alfalfa or red clover sprouts and/or lettuce. Avoid having more than one sandwich on any one day.

FRESH VEGETABLE JUICE COCKTAIL

Makes 1 large serving. *10 Min.*

This is an added plus for the efficiency of the program. Feel free to have it any day you desire before lunch or dinner. Drink it slowly, and allow 10 minutes to pass before eating your meal. If you don't have a juicer, seek out a natural food store that carries fresh juices or makes them to order.

8	large carrots
1	stalk celery
¼	small beet
1	medium tomato
1	small red or green pepper
1	small handful spinach *or* fresh parsley

The carrots and celery are basic. You may add any other vegetables, but approximately one third–two thirds of the juice is *always* carrot. Cut bitter ends off carrots. It is not necessary to pare them. Discard celery leaves. Run all vegetables through juicer.

PERFECT CREAMY CAULIFLOWER SOUP

Serves 4. *35 Min.*

2	tablespoons butter
1	tablespoon olive oil
1	medium onion, coarsely chopped
6–8	scallions, chopped
1	clove garlic, minced
2	stalks celery, chopped
2	medium cauliflower, cored and coarsely chopped
½	teaspoon sea salt
½	teaspoon curry powder (optional)
⅛	teaspoon fresh ground black pepper
½	teaspoon dried thyme[1]
1	teaspoon dried basil

[1]I am not recommending fresh herbs here or in most of the recipes to follow. Cooking with fresh herbs changes the recipe considerably, and the variation between dried and fresh differs for each herb. Also, in most

1 teaspoon dried savory *or* marjoram
6 cups water
2 tablespoons white miso (preferable to vegetable bouillon because it will not turn the soup dark)
⅛ teaspoon fresh ground nutmeg (optional)

In heavy soup kettle, melt butter. Add oil. Add onion, scallions, and garlic. Add celery and cauliflower. Add seasonings. Mix well and cook, uncovered, over medium heat for several minutes, stirring frequently. Add water and miso. Bring to a boil. Simmer, covered, over medium heat for 15 minutes or until cauliflower is tender. Remove cover and cool slightly. Purée in small increments in blender until smooth and creamy. Reheat, adding fresh ground nutmeg, if desired.

POTATO BOATS

Serves 2–4, depending on size of potatoes. *1 Hr 20 Min.*

If you liked those improperly combined baked potatoes with cheese stuffing, try this terrific alternative!

2 large Idaho *or* russet potatoes
1 pound banana squash, approximately ½–¾ cup
¼ cup butter, melted
¼ teaspoon cumin (optional)
1 teaspoon sea salt, seasoned salt, or salt-free seasoning
Sweet Hungarian paprika
2 teaspoons butter, melted

---

areas of the country, there is a short season for fresh herbs, while dried are readily available year-round. I am endeavoring to keep these recipes *simple* and easy to prepare for working women and men, and I would rather avoid the fresh herb complication. In a few instances, I *do* recommend *fresh* herbs, and then I give the specific amounts.

Bake potatoes in preheated 425-degree oven until soft, about 60 minutes. While potatoes are baking, cut skin from squash. Cut squash into small cubes and place in vegetable steamer, covered, over boiling water for 15 minutes or until very soft.

Cool potatoes slightly. Cut them in half while still warm and gently scrape pulp from skin, taking care not to tear skin.

Combine squash, potato pulp, ¼ cup melted butter, cumin, and sea salt with potato masher or in food processor until you have a creamy yellow purée.

Heap potato-squash mixture into empty potato shells. Brush with 2 teaspoons melted butter and sprinkle with paprika. Place under broiler for 10 minutes or until lightly browned.

EASY ROAST CHICKEN

55 Min.

1 small fryer or broiler
Fresh ground black pepper
Sea salt

Preheat oven to 425 degrees. Rub chicken inside and out with sea salt and pepper. Roast in oven for 45–55 minutes, basting frequently with its drippings. Chicken will be golden brown and very juicy, and leg will move easily when it is ready.

GARLIC STRING BEANS

Serves 2. *40 Min.*

2 tablespoons olive oil
1 teaspoon garlic, minced

- 4 cups fresh *or* frozen string beans, cut into 2-inch pieces *or* julienned
- ½ teaspoon dried thyme
- ½ teaspoon sea salt, seasoned salt, *or* salt-free seasoning
- Fresh ground black pepper
- 2 cups water
- 2 teaspoons Gayelord Hauser Natural Vegetable Broth *or* 1 vegetable bouillon
- Squeeze of fresh lemon juice

In large heavy saucepan, heat oil. Add garlic and beans, and sauté over high heat to sear beans, stirring frequently so they do not burn. Add thyme, sea salt, and pepper to taste. Add water and vegetable bouillon. Bring to a boil, cover tightly, reduce heat to medium-low, and simmer for 20–30 minutes or until beans are tender when pierced with tip of sharp knife. Add more water, if necessary. Frozen beans will take only half the time. Add squeeze of lemon juice, and toss well.

French Green Salad

Serves 2. *15 Min.*

- 1 head lettuce – butter, limestone, *or* red leaf
- 1 cup arugula, coarsely chopped (optional)
- 3 tablespoons olive oil
- 1 tablespoon fresh lemon juice
- ¼–½ teaspoon sea salt, seasoned salt, *or* salt-free seasoning
- Fresh ground black pepper

Wash and thoroughly dry lettuce and arugula. Break lettuce into bite-size pieces, discarding center stalk of each leaf. Combine lettuce and arugula in large bowl.

Add oil, and toss well. Add lemon juice, sea salt, and pepper to taste, and toss gently so lettuce does not become wilted.

MAIN-COURSE SALAD DAY

DAY TWO – TUESDAY

This is your first MAIN-COURSE SALAD DAY. You will be having fruit at breakfast and at lunch, and any fresh juices you desire, with a main-course salad in the evening. Remember that tomato, avocado, and cucumber are vegetable fruit, so these may be included in the fruits you eat during the day. If you do have the Vegetable-fruit Platter at lunch, give the avocado one to two hours to digest before having other fruit. Tomato and cucumber mixed do not require additional time to digest. They are very high in water content. You may also eat raw vegetables, such as celery and carrots, but allow one to two hours to pass before you eat fruit after these and avocado. Plain raw vegetables, being very high in water content, will not remain for very long in the stomach.

BREAKFAST:

Same as Day One.

LUNCH:

Continue on fruit, *or* you may have the Vegetable-fruit Platter.*

DINNER:

Fresh Vegetable Juice Cocktail (see page 241), *or*
1 papaya, *or* fresh pineapple spears
Mediterranean Rice Salad*

VEGETABLE-FRUIT PLATTER

Serves 1. *5 Min.*

1 *or* 2	medium tomatoes, sliced
1	small cucumber *or* 2 pickling cukes, peeled and sliced
½	large avocado, peeled and sliced
	Dulse flakes *or* salt-free seasoning (optional)

Arrange vegetable fruits on platter, and sprinkle with dulse flakes or salt-free seasoning.

MEDITERRANEAN RICE SALAD

Serves 2. *30-60 Min. (depending on rice used)*

1	cup long-grain brown rice *or* basmati rice (see recipe following)
1	tablespoon olive oil
4	medium zucchini, cut into ¼-inch slices
1–2	tablespoons water
1	teaspoon dried basil
1	teaspoon dried oregano
4	cups lettuce – iceberg, butter, red leaf, *or* romaine (*or* any combination of these)
2	cups spinach *or* arugula, coarsely chopped
1	cup alfalfa sprouts
½	cup pimento-stuffed green olives, sliced

Prepare the rice.

Basmati rice is particularly special in this recipe, but if it is not available, long-grain brown rice is a good substitute.

1	cup long-grain brown rice
2½	cups water
1	tablespoon unrefined safflower oil

In a large saucepan, combine all ingredients, bring to a boil, stir gently. Simmer, covered, over low heat for 40 minutes. Remove from heat without lifting cover. Allow to sit for 10 minutes before lifting cover.

OR

1	cup basmati rice
2	cups water
1	tablespoon unrefined safflower oil

In a large saucepan, combine all ingredients, bring to a boil, stir gently. Simmer, covered, over low heat for 20 minutes. Lift cover immediately, and fluff with fork.

Prepare the zucchini.

Heat oil in wok or large skillet. Add zucchini slices, and toss in oil. Sprinkle with water and continue tossing for several minutes until zucchini turns a brighter color. Add basil and oregano. Toss gently and set aside.

GARLIC HERB DRESSING:

1	clove garlic, minced *or* crushed
5	tablespoons olive oil
2	tablespoons fresh lemon *or* lime juice
½	teaspoon dried chervil
½	teaspoon dried marjoram
¼	teaspoon dried mint

½ teaspoon dried thyme
⅛ teaspoon dried tarragon
½ teaspoon sea salt, seasoned salt, *or* salt-free seasoning
Fresh ground black pepper

Prepare the dressing.
Place all ingredients in bowl, and whip with fork or whisk, or combine ingredients in blender or food processor.

Assemble the salad.
Wash and dry lettuce, and break into bite-size pieces, and combine in large bowl with spinach or arugula and sprouts. Add rice, zucchini, olives, and dressing. Toss well to combine all flavors.

Remember, if you are hungry, a fruit snack at least three hours after dinner is very much to your advantage, since the added water content will aid elimination on the following day.

DAY THREE – WEDNESDAY

BREAKFAST:

Same as Day One.

LUNCH:

Fresh fruit *or* carrot juice (optional)
Nut Butter Dip* with raw vegetables, *or* Energy Salad (with Light Dressing or dressing of your choice)
(see pages 238–239)

DINNER:

Country Corn Chowder*
New York Goodwich*
Spinach–Sprout Salad*

NUT BUTTER DIP

1 Min.

In this recipe, unsalted raw almond, cashew, sesame, or sunflower seed butters are best. Peanut butter may be substituted, if desired.

¼ cup nut butter, smooth *or* chunky
¼ cup water

Whip nut butter and water with fork until light, creamy dipping sauce forms. Use as dip for celery, carrots, zucchini, green or red peppers, jicama, raw cauliflower or broccoli, fennel, or sliced Jerusalem artichokes.

COUNTRY CORN CHOWDER

Serves 4. *35 Min.*

6 cups water
6 medium all-purpose potatoes, peeled and cubed
1 medium onion, chopped
2 cloves garlic, minced
1 stalk celery, chopped
2 vegetable bouillon *or* 1 vegetable bouillon and 1 tablespoon light miso
⅛ teaspoon dried sage
½ teaspoon dried thyme
½ teaspoon dried oregano

½ teaspoon sea salt (optional)
½ teaspoon seasoned salt *or* salt-free seasoning
Fresh ground pepper to taste
3–4 cups fresh *or* frozen corn
1 tablespoon butter
¼ cup green pepper, minced
½ cup scallions, minced
¼ cup heavy cream (optional)
1 tablespoon fresh dill, minced (optional)

Bring water to a boil. Add potatoes, onion, garlic, and celery. Return water to a boil and add bouillon and seasonings. Cover and simmer over medium heat for 15–20 minutes or until potatoes are tender but not mushy. Cool slightly. Remove 2 cups of potatoes from stock and set aside. Blend remaining chowder in small increments. Reheat over low heat. Add corn and reserved potatoes. Simmer, stirring to insure that chowder does not stick, for 5 minutes. Melt butter in a small skillet. Add green pepper and scallions. Sauté until vegetables turn a bright green, approximately 3 minutes. Stir into simmering chowder. Add cream and dill, if desired. Adjust seasonings.

NEW YORK GOODWICH

Serves 1. *25 Min.*

Believe it or not, this conglomeration of vegetables results in an absolutely delectable 'handwich' – something that can really become a great addiction! Seven hundred and fifty people devoured 1,600 of these at one of our seminars on the Queen Mary *in Long Beach, California. It was a new experience, and they loved it!*

- 1 cup broccoli
- ½ cup cauliflower (optional)
- 2 tablespoons carrot, finely grated
- 2 tablespoons red cabbage, finely grated
- 2 tablespoons yellow squash, finely grated
- ¼ cup Barbecued Onions (see below) (optional)
- 1 whole-wheat tortilla, chapati, or pita
- 1 tablespoon mayonnaise
- 3 thin slivers dill pickle
- ½ cup lettuce, finely shredded
- ½ cup alfalfa sprouts
- 2 slices avocado (optional)
- Dash of sea salt, Spike, *or* salt-free seasoning (optional)

Prepare the vegetables.

Cut broccoli into thin lengths, using only florets and upper portion of stalk. Break cauliflower into tiny florets. Place broccoli and cauliflower in vegetable steamer, covered, over boiling water for 5 minutes or until vegetables are tender when pierced with tip of sharp knife. Combine carrot, cabbage, and squash, and mix thoroughly.

BARBECUED ONIONS FOR GOODWICH:

- 2 teaspoons safflower oil
- 1 small white onion, sliced
- ½ tablespoon Hain or Robbie's barbecue sauce

Prepare the Barbecued Onions.

In a small skillet, heat oil. Add onion, and sauté until it begins to soften. Add barbecue sauce, and continue sautéing, stirring frequently, until onion is thoroughly wilted. Makes enough for three or four Goodwiches. Leftover Barbecued Onions are delicious in any vegetable soup.

Assemble the Goodwich.
In hot *dry* skillet, heat tortilla or chapati, turning from one side to the other until soft but *not crisp*. Place on large sheet of plastic wrap. If using pita, heat in oven for a few minutes to soften it, and cut a sliver from top so pocket opens easily. Combine all other ingredients, mix well, and stuff into pocket.

Spread tortilla with mayonnaise. Add a line of broccoli down center. Crumble cauliflower and place a line of it on broccoli. Add a line of pickle, a line of grated vegetables, a line of Barbecued Onions. Top with lettuce, sprouts, and avocado. Sprinkle with Spike, if desired. Roll tortilla tightly, crepe-style, around vegetables. Wrap tightly in plastic wrap until ready to serve. This Goodwich will keep for two–three days in the refrigerator (if you hide it from your friends and family!). Cut it in half and push plastic wrap partially down, but leave one end closed to catch the drippy sauces. YUM!

SPINACH–SPROUT SALAD

Serves 2. *15 Min.*

2 cups lettuce, chopped
2 cups spinach, chopped
2 cups alfalfa sprouts
1 cup assorted sprouts – lentil, mung bean, aduki, radish, fenugreek, pea, red clover, wheat berry
1 cup cucumber, peeled and cubed
1 medium tomato, sliced
1 cup arugula, chopped (optional)
2 tablespoons olive oil
2 teaspoons fresh lemon juice
2 teaspoons Bragg Liquid Aminos, soy sauce, *or* ½ teaspoon Dijon mustard

Combine vegetables and sprouts in large bowl. Add oil and toss. Add lemon juice and Liquid Aminos or soy sauce or mustard, and toss again.

DAY FOUR – THURSDAY

BREAKFAST:

Same as Day One.

LUNCH:

Fresh fruit *or* carrot juice (optional)
Nuts and Cukes,* *or* Energy Salad (see page 238)
with cottage cheese, if desired

DINNER:

Fresh Vegetable Juice Cocktail (see page 241)
Stew for Two*
Caesar Salad*
Curried Cabbage*

NUTS AND CUKES

2 Min.

½–1 cup raw almonds, pecans, walnuts, Brazil nuts, *or* filberts
1 medium cucumber, peeled and cut into spears

Make sure nuts are raw. If they have been roasted, they are unusable in the body and only toxify it. Nuts and Cukes may not *sound* like much of a lunch, but it is a very satisfying finger-food meal, which takes a while to eat because nuts must be chewed well. The flavors are *very* complementary – the nutritional benefits are impeccable! This is the *perfect* way to eat nuts.

STEW FOR TWO

Serves 2. *40 Min.*

8	tiny new potatoes
3	large carrots
2–3	tablespoons butter
1	small onion, chopped
1	stalk celery, chopped
4	broccoli stalks without florets, peeled and cut into ½-inch pieces
2	small zucchini, sliced
1	cup frozen lima beans (optional)
½	cup frozen peas (optional)
¼	teaspoon celery seed
¼	teaspoon dried sage
¼	teaspoon dried marjoram
½	teaspoon sea salt, seasoned salt, *or* salt-free seasoning
1	Morga or Hügli vegetable bouillon *or* 2 teaspoons Hauser Natural Vegetable Broth
1–2	cups water

Place potatoes and carrots, whole, in vegetable steamer, covered, over boiling water for 15 minutes. Cut carrots into ½-inch slices. Peel potatoes and cut into 1-inch cubes. Set aside. Melt butter in large heavy saucepan. Add potatoes, carrots, onion, celery, broccoli, salt, herbs, bouillon, and water. Bring to a boil. Then simmer, covered, for 5 minutes. Add zucchini, lima beans and peas. Return to boil, cover, and simmer for 10 minutes, stirring occasionally. Kids love to dip whole-grain buttered toast into this delightful stew.

CAESAR SALAD

Serves 2. *15 Min.*

1 clove garlic
3 tablespoons olive oil
1–2 tablespoons fresh lemon juice
1 teaspoon Dijon mustard
1 sheet nori (pressed seaweed, available in natural food stores or in Asian food section of your supermarket) (optional)
¼ teaspoon sea salt, seasoned salt, *or* salt-free seasoning
1 small head romaine
1 cup Garlic Croutons (see below)
Fresh ground black pepper

Place garlic in large bowl and crush with fork. Add oil and stir briskly. Discard garlic. Add lemon juice and mustard, and combine with fork. Holding nori in your hand, toast it over hot burner (gas or electric) for 1–2 seconds on each side, until it turns from black to green. Crumble into pieces and mix into dressing. Add sea salt, and whip dressing. Wash and thoroughly dry lettuce. Break into bite-size pieces, discarding heaviest part of stalk. Add to bowl, and toss thoroughly in dressing. Add Garlic Croutons (see below) and pepper to taste. Toss again.

GARLIC CROUTONS:
Serves 1–2. *10 Min.*

These are easy to make and far superior to the packaged variety.

1 slice whole-grain bread
2 teaspoons butter
1 clove garlic, crushed *or* cut into 2 or 3 pieces

Cut bread into small cubes. In small skillet, melt butter. Add garlic. Sauté briefly to flavor butter. Discard garlic. Add bread and sauté, turning frequently, until crisp. Add cubes to salad, soup, or vegetable dishes.

CURRIED CABBAGE

Serves 3–4. *12 Min.*

1	tablespoon safflower oil
2	teaspoons mustard seeds
1	teaspoon turmeric
1	small white onion, quartered and sliced thin
1	small head cabbage, cored, quartered, and sliced thin
½	teaspoon sea salt
2	tablespoons fresh lemon *or* lime juice

In large skillet, heat oil. Add mustard seeds and turmeric, and allow to sizzle for a moment. Add onion, and sauté for several minutes, stirring frequently. Add cabbage and salt, and mix thoroughly. Cook, uncovered, over medium heat, stirring continuously, until cabbage begins to wilt. Sprinkle with lemon or lime juice.

MAIN-COURSE SALAD DAY

DAY FIVE – FRIDAY

BREAKFAST:

Same as Day One.

LUNCH:

Continue on fruit and juice all day, *or* you may have the Vegetable-fruit Platter (see page 247).

DINNER:

Fresh Vegetable Juice Cocktail (see page 241),
or ½ cantaloupe, *or* 1 whole grapefruit
Curried Chicken Salad*

CURRIED CHICKEN SALAD

Makes 1 very large or 2 moderate-sized salads.

25 Min. (plus preparation time for chicken)

- 4 cups butter lettuce, washed, dried, and broken into bite-size pieces
- 2 cups spinach, coarsely chopped
- ½ cup alfalfa sprouts
- ¼ cup arugula *or* fresh cilantro, chopped (optional)
- 2 cups Easy Roast Chicken, skinned and shredded (see page 244), *or* any broiled, steamed, or barbecued chicken
- 2 cups asparagus
- ½ cup carrots, slivered

Prepare the salad.

In large bowl, combine lettuce, spinach, sprouts, and arugula or cilantro. Break and discard tough ends from asparagus, and cut into 1-inch diagonals. Drop asparagus into boiling water. Boil for 3–4 minutes or until it turns bright green. Remove from boiling water, and place immediately under cold water. Pour boiling water over carrots and allow them to blanch for 1–2 minutes. Drain. Add chicken, asparagus, and carrots to salad greens.

CURRIED MAYONNAISE DRESSING:

- 2 tablespoons olive oil
- 1 tablespoon fresh lemon juice
- 1–2 tablespoons mayonnaise
- 1 teaspoon honey
- ½ teaspoon curry powder
- ½ teaspoon dried basil *or* 2 teaspoons fresh basil, minced
- 1 teaspoon scallions, minced
- ¼ teaspoon sea salt (optional)
- Fresh ground black pepper

Prepare the dressing.

In small bowl, combine oil, lemon juice, mayonnaise, and honey. Whisk until creamy. Add curry powder, basil, scallions, and sea salt. Whisk again. Pour over salad. Season with pepper to taste.

DAY SIX – SATURDAY

BREAKFAST:

Same as Day One.

LUNCH:

Fresh fruit *or* carrot juice (optional)
Energy Salad (see page 238), *or* Cauliflower Toastie*

DINNER:

Harvest Soup* and Hot Buttered Corn Tortillas,* *or*
Carrot Hash Browns*
Teriyaki Broccoli*
Tangy Green Coleslaw*

CAULIFLOWER TOASTIE

Serves 1. *20 Min.*

A simple toastie maker, inexpensive to purchase at your local hardware store, is the best tool for toasties. If you don't have one, spread the filling on buttered toast. Toastie makers (my term) used to be called toastites. They are now called snack, sandwich, or pie cookers, made by Aluma, available in hardware stores for under ten dollars. They have a 2-part folding griddle, round or square, the size of a piece of bread, with a long handle. Place bread and fillings inside, close and set on a burner, turning so both sides cook.

1 cup cauliflower, steamed
1–2 tablespoons mayonnaise
¼ teaspoon Dijon mustard (optional)
¼ teaspoon sea salt, seasoned salt, *or* salt-free seasoning
1 teaspoon celery *or* water chestnuts, chopped (optional)
2 slices whole-grain bread
1 tablespoon butter
½ cup alfalfa sprouts *or* lettuce, shredded
1 tablespoon carrots, shredded

Mash cauliflower, mixing in mayonnaise, mustard, and sea salt. Add celery or water chestnuts, and mix well. Butter bread. Spread cauliflower mixture on unbuttered side of one slice of bread. Sprinkle with sprouts or lettuce and carrots. Cover with second slice of bread, buttered side facing out. Place sandwich in toastie maker. Heat over high flame until bread is golden and toasted, and filling is warm, approximately 3 minutes each side.

Harvest Soup

Serves 8. *55 Min.*

9 cups water
1 large white onion, coarsely chopped
2 large cloves garlic, minced
2 stalks celery, coarsely chopped
1 medium celery root (celeriac), peeled and cubed (optional)
2 cups banana squash, cubed
1 small cauliflower, cored and cut into 1-inch florets
4 medium carrots, peeled and cut into ½-inch cubes

4	medium zucchini, cut into ¼-inch slices
4	medium golden zucchini *or* summer squash, cut into ¼-inch slices
3	medium White Rose potatoes, peeled, halved, and cut into ¼-inch slices
1	small head savoy cabbage, cored, quartered, and sliced thin
½	teaspoon dried thyme
½	teaspoon dried basil
½	teaspoon dried summer savory
2	tablespoons white miso *or* 2 vegetable bouillon
1	teaspoon sea salt (optional)
	Dash of cinnamon
	Dash of nutmeg
2	tablespoons fresh lemon juice

In heavy soup kettle, bring water to a boil. Add all ingredients except lemon juice. Return to boil. Simmer for 30 minutes, stirring frequently to break up squash and form thick stock. Stir in lemon juice at end of cooking. This soup can be made in large quantities, because it is a great leftover.

Hot Buttered Corn Tortillas

Serves 4. *8 Min.*

8	corn tortillas
2	tablespoons butter

Heat tortillas one at a time in hot *dry* skillet, turning from one side to the other until soft but not crisp. After heating one, place a dollop of butter in center, and stack another hot tortilla on top. Place stack of tortillas in covered casserole to keep them warm and soft; otherwise they dry out. To eat, you can cut in wedges like a pie, or pick up individual tortillas and roll them, which is the more traditional way of eating them.

Carrot Hash Browns

Serves 3. *30 Min.*

- 2 tablespoons butter
- 1 teaspoon safflower oil
- 3 medium carrots, peeled and finely grated
- 3 medium all-purpose potatoes, peeled and finely grated
- ½ small white onion, finely grated
- ½ teaspoon sea salt (optional)

In large skillet, melt butter and oil. Add carrots, potatoes, and onions. Add seasoning. Sauté until browned on one side. Flip over, and sauté on second side until browned. Break apart into small chunks, or serve in wedges cut from the round.

Teriyaki Broccoli

Serves 3. *15 Min.*

This is a delicious dish that gives you an opportunity to use up some of your leftover broccoli stalks.

- 3 or 4 thick broccoli stalks without florets
- 1 tablespoon sesame *or* safflower oil
- 1–2 cloves garlic, minced
- 2 tablespoons tamari
- Squeeze of fresh lemon juice (optional)

Use carrot peeler to remove thick skin from outside of stalks. Cut stalks lengthwise in thin slices. In large skillet, heat oil. Add garlic, sautéing briefly. Add broccoli. Sauté 3–5 minutes over medium-high heat, until tender. Toss in tamari and lemon.

TANGY GREEN COLESLAW

Serves 3. *15 Min.*

- ½ small head cabbage
- 2 tablespoons fresh dill, chopped
- 2 tablespoons fresh parsley, chopped
- ½ cup sour cream
- Juice of 1 small lemon
- ½ teaspoon dulse flakes (optional)
- ½ teaspoon sea salt, seasoned salt, *or* salt-free seasoning
- Fresh ground black pepper

Grate cabbage, cut into thin strips, or chop finely. In large bowl, combine cabbage, dill, and parsley. Blend together sour cream and lemon juice. Pour over cabbage. Add dulse, sea salt, and pepper to taste. Mix well. (Save leftover coleslaw for Day Nine.)

DAY SEVEN – SUNDAY

BREAKFAST:

Same as Day One, *or* fruit salad of your choice, *or* Strawberry–Kiwi Salad* with Fruit Dip*

LUNCH:

Fresh fruit *or* carrot juice (optional)
Harvest Soup (see page 261) and salad of your choice with dressing of your choice, *or* Cuke-a-tillas*

DINNER:

Fresh Vegetable Juice Cocktail (see page 241)
Shepherd's Pie*
Sweet Basil Carrots*
Salade Parisienne with Asparagus*

STRAWBERRY–KIWI SALAD

Serves 2. *10 Min.*

- 2 oranges, peeled and sliced across the sections
- 2 cups strawberries, sliced
- 2 large kiwi fruit, peeled and sliced
- 1 small banana, peeled and sliced
- 1 tablespoon currants (optional)

On small platter make a bed of orange wheels. In a large bowl, combine strawberries, kiwi fruit, and banana. Add currants. Mix gently and mound on oranges. Make Fruit Dip (see page 266) and pour it over salad, or serve separately.

FRUIT DIP

3 Min. each

Here are 5 different fruit dip suggestions. There are many more possibilities.

Purée in blender or food processor:

1) ½ papaya, ¼ cup fresh orange juice, and ¼ teaspoon nutmeg; *or*
2) 1 persimmon and 1 banana; *or*
3) 1 banana and ½ cup strawberries; *or*
4) ½ cup fresh orange or apple juice, and 6–8 pitted dates; *or*
5) ½ cup pineapple cubes and 1 banana

Serve on or with fruit salad.

CUKE-A-TILLAS

Serving suggestion: *5 Min.*
3 Cuke-a-tillas per person.

Corn tortillas
Mayonnaise *or* butter
Cucumber spears
Alfalfa sprouts *or* lettuce, shredded
Spike, Vegesal, *or* Parsley Patch Mexican Seasoning (salt-free)

Peel cucumber and cut into thin spears 5–6 inches long. Heat 1 tortilla in hot *dry* skillet, turning from one side to the other until soft but *not crisp.* Spread hot tortilla with mayonnaise. Arrange a line of 2–3 cucumber spears down center of tortilla. Top with sprouts or lettuce and seasoning. Roll tightly.

Shepherd's Pie

Serves 4–6. *90 Min.*

STUFFING:

- ½ cup butter
- 1 medium white onion, finely chopped
- 1 shallot, finely chopped
- 1 cup celery, finely chopped
- ¼ cup scallions, minced
- 8 cups whole-grain bread cubes (½-inch cubes), preferably stale
- 2 teaspoons ground sage
- ½ teaspoon dried marjoram
- ½ teaspoon dried thyme
- ½ teaspoon celery seed
- ¼ teaspoon paprika
- ½ teaspoon sea salt
- Fresh ground black pepper
- 1 tablespoon fresh parsley, minced
- 1 Morga or Hügli vegetable bouillon
- 2 cups boiling water

MASHED POTATO CRUST:

- 8–10 small White Rose potatoes, peeled and cut into 2-inch cubes (8–10 cups)
- 1 stalk celery with leaves
- 1 bay leaf
- 1 large clove garlic
- 3 tablespoons butter
- ¼ cup raw *or* heavy cream
- ½ teaspoon sea salt, seasoned salt, *or* salt-free seasoning
- Fresh ground white pepper

Peel potatoes and place in large kettle of cold water. Add celery, bay leaf, and garlic. Bring to a boil, cover, and simmer for 20–30 minutes or until potatoes are tender.

While potatoes are cooking, prepare stuffing. In large heavy saucepan, melt butter. Add onion, shallot, celery, and scallions. Sauté until vegetables begin to soften. Add bread cubes, sage, marjoram, thyme, celery seed, paprika, sea salt, parsley and pepper. Mix well. Dissolve 1 vegetable bouillon in 2 cups boiling water. Add to stuffing, and mix well. Steam, covered, over *very* low heat, stirring frequently, for 15 minutes.

Preheat oven to 375 degrees. Prepare mashed potatoes. In small skillet, melt butter, and add cream. Heat until hot, but do not boil. Remove bay leaf and garlic, and place potatoes in food processor or mash by hand, mixing in butter-cream mixture. Add sea salt and pepper to taste and whip thoroughly.

Place stuffing in oven-proof casserole. Top with mashed potatoes. Bake in oven for 30–45 minutes or until potatoes have formed a golden crust. Prepare Mushroom Cream Gravy (see below) while pie bakes.

MUSHROOM CREAM GRAVY:

- 2 tablespoons butter
- 1 shallot, minced
- 1 pound mushrooms, sliced
- 2 tablespoons butter
- 2 tablespoons flour
- 1½ cups water
- 2 vegetable bouillon
- 2 tablespoons raw *or* heavy cream
- ½ teaspoon sea salt
- ¼ teaspoon garlic crystals *or* garlic salt

In large heavy skillet, melt 2 tablespoons butter. Add shallot and mushrooms, and sauté until mushrooms are soft and have released a dark brown juice. Remove mushrooms from pan with slotted spoon. Pour juice into measuring cup and reserve.

In same skillet, melt 2 tablespoons butter. Add flour, and stir with whisk to combine. Add mushroom liquid, and continue stirring with whisk as gravy thickens. Slowly add water, whisking continuously, and add bouillon. Whisk to dissolve bouillon. Add cream, salt, and garlic. At this point mushrooms may be added to gravy, or you may serve it plain over Shepherd's Pie.

SWEET BASIL CARROTS

Serves 4–6. *25 Min.*

12	medium carrots, peeled
3	tablespoons sweet butter
2	tablespoons pure maple syrup
1–2	teaspoons fresh basil
¼	teaspoon sea salt

Cut carrots into ⅛-inch slices or run through slicer of food processor. Place them in vegetable steamer, covered, over boiling water for 10 minutes until tender but not mushy. Remove from heat and set aside. Carrots may be steamed well in advance and combined with other ingredients immediately before serving. In large heavy saucepan, melt butter. Add maple syrup, carrots, basil, and sea salt. Stir well to coat carrots thoroughly with butter sauce.

Salade Parisienne with Asparagus

Serves 4. *15 Min.*

1	head butter lettuce
½	head red leaf lettuce
½	pound fresh *or* frozen asparagus

Prepare the salad.

Wash lettuce, dry thoroughly, and break into bite-size pieces, discarding heavy center stalk. Break and discard heavy ends from asparagus, and plunge, whole, into boiling water for 3–5 minutes or until bright green and tender-crisp. Remove from water, drain well, and cut into 1½-inch pieces. Combine with lettuce.

FRENCH DRESSING:

3	tablespoons olive oil
1	tablespoon fresh lemon juice
½	teaspoon Dijon mustard
	Sea salt (optional)
1	clove garlic, halved
	Fresh ground black pepper

Prepare the dressing.

Place oil, lemon juice, mustard, and sea salt to taste in measuring cup. Skewer garlic on fork, and whip dressing with garlic fork. Pour over salad. Add pepper to taste, and toss well.

MAIN-COURSE SALAD DAY

DAY EIGHT – MONDAY

BREAKFAST:

Same as Day One.

LUNCH:

Continue on fruit and juice all day, *or* you may have the Vegetable-fruit Platter (see page 247).

DINNER:

Fresh Vegetable Juice Cocktail (see page 241) *or*
½ cantaloupe *or* ½ honeydew melon
Award-winning Potato-lovers' Salad*

AWARD-WINNING POTATO LOVERS' SALAD

Serves 2. *35 Min.*

- 6 tiny new potatoes (red-skinned)
- 2 tablespoons butter
- ½ teaspoon sea salt, seasoned salt, *or* salt-free seasoning
- ¼ teaspoon sweet Hungarian paprika
- 2 cups broccoli florets (leave 2 inches of stems attached)
- 4 cups head lettuce, washed, dried, and broken into bite-size pieces
- 2 cups spinach, coarsely chopped

1 cup alfalfa sprouts
1 cup red cabbage, finely sliced or shredded

Prepare the salad.

Place potatoes whole and unpeeled in vegetable steamer, covered, over boiling water for 20 minutes or until almost tender. While potatoes are steaming, prepare broccoli, greens, and dressing. Remove potatoes from heat and cut into ½-inch cubes (peeling is optional). Place in large bowl and set aside. Melt butter in small saucepan. Pour butter over potatoes, and toss well. Add sea salt and paprika, and mix well. Place potatoes in one layer on cookie sheet. Place at highest shelf position in preheated broiler. Broil for 5–10 minutes.

While potatoes are broiling, steam broccoli whole for 5–7 minutes or until just tender and bright green. Remove from heat immediately, and set aside to cool.

Place lettuce and spinach in large bowl, and add sprouts, separated so they don't clump. Add cabbage. Cut broccoli lengthwise into thin slivers. Add to greens.

CREAMY DRESSING:

1 large clove garlic
2 tablespoons fresh lemon *or* lime juice
¼–½ teaspoon sea salt (optional)
¼ cup olive oil
½ teaspoon dried oregano
¼ teaspoon dried thyme
1–2 tablespoons mayonnaise
Fresh ground black pepper (optional)

Prepare the dressing.

Peel garlic and crush (if you like a heavy garlic flavor) or cut in half (if you prefer a milder salad). Place garlic in measuring cup, and pierce with fork. Add lemon or lime juice, salt, olive oil, and herbs. Add mayonnaise, and whip dressing with garlic fork until thick and creamy. Pour dressing over salad, and toss well.

Complete the salad.
Remove potatoes from broiler. Add to salad. Season with pepper, if desired. Toss well.

DAY NINE – TUESDAY

BREAKFAST:

Same as Day One.

LUNCH:

Fresh fruit *or* carrot juice (optional)
Energy Salad (see page 238) *or* Great Guacamole*
with corn chips and celery stalks

DINNER:

Fresh Vegetable Juice Cocktail (see page 241)
Crusty Butter-crumb Vegetables,*
or buttered whole-grain toast
Blue Ribbon Split Pea Soup*
Tangy Green Coleslaw (see page 244)

Great Guacamole

Serves 1–2. *5 Min.*

1 avocado
½ teaspoon Spike *or* Parsley Patch Mexican Seasoning (salt-free)
½ teaspoon cumin
½ teaspoon dried oregano

Cut avocado in half, remove seed, and scoop out pulp, reserving seed. In small bowl, mash with fork, mixing in seasonings. Whip with fork until creamy. If you are not going to serve guacamole immediately, return seed to bowl to prevent discoloration, cover tightly, and refrigerate until ready to use. Serve as dip for natural corn chips, celery stalks, or other raw vegetables.

Crusty Butter-Crumb Vegetables

Serves 4. *25 Min.*

1 medium cauliflower, cored and broken into small florets
¼ head red cabbage, cored and shredded
6 medium carrots, cut into slices or matchsticks, or diced
2 medium yellow squash, cut into ½-inch cubes
2 cups bok choy greens, shredded

Prepare the vegetables.
Place cauliflower, cabbage, carrots, and squash in vegetable steamer, covered, over boiling water for 10 minutes or until tender. Add bok choy greens for last minute of steaming to wilt them.

BUTTER-CRUMB TOPPING:

- 2 tablespoons butter
- 1 clove garlic, minced
- 4 slices whole-grain bread

Prepare the topping.
In large heavy skillet, melt butter. Add garlic and sauté for flavor. In food processor or blender, process bread to a medium consistency. Toss bread crumbs in garlic butter until all butter has been absorbed and crumbs are evenly coated.

- 1 tablespoon butter
- ½ teaspoon Spike
- ¼ teaspoon sea salt
- Fresh ground black pepper
- 2 tablespoons butter

Assemble the casserole.
Preheat oven to 500 degrees. In large bowl, toss steamed vegetables with 1 tablespoon butter, Spike, and sea salt. Add pepper, if desired, and ½ cup butter-crumb topping. Mix well. Spread vegetables in shallow oven-proof casserole. Top with remaining crumb topping. Dot with 2 tablespoons butter. Bake in oven for 5 minutes. Any leftover casserole can be added to soups, used in vegetable toasties, or rolled in hot chapatis.

BLUE RIBBON SPLIT PEA SOUP

Serves 8. *1 Hr 40 Min.*

- 2 tablespoons butter
- 1 tablespoon safflower oil
- 1 cup carrots, coarsely chopped
- 1 cup celery, coarsely chopped
- 1½ cups onion, coarsely chopped
- 1 large clove garlic, minced
- 2 cups cabbage, finely shredded
- 10 cups water
- 2 cups green split peas
- 1 teaspoon dried basil
- 1 teaspoon dried thyme
- 1 teaspoon dried marjoram
- ½ teaspoon dried oregano
- ½ teaspoon dried summer savory
- ⅛ teaspoon dried sage
- ⅛ teaspoon dried tarragon
- ¼ teaspoon celery seed
- ¼ teaspoon ground coriander
- ½ teaspoon sea salt (optional)
- ¼ teaspoon seasoned salt *or* salt-free seasoning
- Fresh ground pepper to taste
- 1 vegetable bouillon
- 4 tablespoons fresh parsley, minced

Heat the butter and oil together in a large soup kettle. Add the carrots, celery, onion, garlic, and cabbage and sauté, stirring frequently, for several minutes. Add the water, the split peas, the seasonings, and the bouillon. Bring to a boil. Cover and simmer over medium heat for 1½ hours, stirring frequently. Stir in the parsley and adjust the seasonings. This soup freezes beautifully so freeze any left over in an airtight container to be used for another meal.

DAY TEN – WEDNESDAY

BREAKFAST:

Same as Day One.

LUNCH:

Fresh fruit *or* carrot juice (optional)
The Properly Combined Sandwich (see page 239) *or*
Nut Butter Dip and raw vegetables (see page 250), *or*
Nuts and Cukes (see page 254)

DINNER:

Fresh Vegetable Juice Cocktail (see page 241)
Stir-fried Lo Mein with Shredded Vegetables*
Caesar Salad (see page 256; omit croutons, if desired)
Perfect Corn on the Cob*

STIR-FRIED LO MEIN WITH SHREDDED VEGETABLES

Serves 2. *25 Min.*

- 1 tablespoon safflower oil
- 1 teaspoon garlic, minced
- ½ teaspoon fresh ginger (optional)
- 2 cups cabbage, shredded
- 1 cup scallions, cut in long slivers
- 2 cups zucchini, cut into ¼-inch diagonal slices, then slivered into matchsticks
- 1 cup snow peas, shredded

2 cups asparagus *or* broccoli, cut into 1-inch diagonals or thin florets
3 tablespoons safflower oil
4 cups cold cooked noodles (buckwheat soba, jinenjo noodles,[2] De Cecco whole-wheat spaghetti, *or* any other whole-wheat or vegetable noodle)

If using broccoli, presteam for 4 minutes. Heat wok for several minutes while preparing vegetables. Add 1 tablespoon oil and swirl in wok to coat sides. Add garlic and ginger, and immediately add all vegetables. Stir-fry in hot oil, adding 1–2 tablespoons of water if necessary to keep vegetables from scorching. Stir-fry until vegetables turn bright green (just a few minutes), then turn them out on large platter. Wash wok and replace over medium-high heat.

SAUCE:

1 tablespoon tofu sauce *or* tamari
1 teaspoon fresh lemon juice *or* dry sherry
1 tablespoon roasted sesame oil
2 tablespoons Hain barbecue sauce *or* Chinese bean *or* peanut sauce[3]
1 teaspoon honey
1 teaspoon hot curry paste (optional) *or* ½ teaspoon curry powder

In small bowl, combine all ingredients. Mix well, and set aside.

Heat 3 tablespoons oil in hot wok. Add noodles, and stir-fry until warm. Add vegetables and sauce. Toss to combine well. Turn out on large platter.

[2] Spaghetti-like noodles made from wild mountain sweet potatoes, available in Asian markets or natural food stores.
[3] Available in Asian markets.

Perfect Corn on the Cob

Serves 2–4. *7 Min.*

4	ears of corn
	Butter
	Sea salt, seasoned salt, *or* salt-free seasoning

Always store corn in husks in refrigerator. It will keep much better and longer. In soup kettle, bring water to a boil. Add husked corn, and boil for exactly 5 minutes. Remove to platter. Add butter and sea salt.

MAIN-COURSE SALAD DAY

Remember, for any dinner you may substitute the main-course salad of your choice.

DAY ELEVEN – THURSDAY

BREAKFAST:

Same as Day One.

LUNCH:

Fresh fruit *or* carrot juice (optional)
Continue on fruit with a fruit salad *or*
the Vegetable-fruit Platter (see page 247)
Have raw vegetables, if desired.

DINNER:

1 whole grapefruit
Steak-lovers' Salad* (the Texas Salad)

STEAK-LOVERS' SALAD

Serves 2. *40 Min.*

3	cups Garlic String Beans (see page 244)
10–12	ounces steak – porterhouse, filet mignon, flank, or whatever cut you prefer
2	teaspoons safflower oil
1	small red *or* white onion, sliced
4	cups butter lettuce, washed, dried, and broken into bite-size pieces
2	cups spinach, stems removed

3	large mushrooms, sliced or cut into matchsticks

Prepare the salad.
Prepare Garlic String Beans. While beans are cooking, broil steak according to taste. Cut into thin diagonal strips and set aside. Heat oil in small skillet. Sauté onion in oil until tender and beginning to crisp. Place lettuce and spinach in large bowl. Add steak, string beans, onion, and mushrooms.

DIJON DRESSING:

3	tablespoons olive oil
1	tablespoon fresh lemon juice
¾	teaspoon Dijon mustard
½	teaspoon sea salt, seasoned salt, *or* salt-free seasoning (optional)
¼	teaspoon Spike (optional)
	Fresh ground black pepper

Prepare the dressing.
In small bowl, whisk until frothy oil, lemon juice, and mustard. Add sea salt and Spike, if desired. Pour over salad. Add pepper to taste. Toss well.

Have a fruit snack before bed, as long as 4 hours have elapsed since dinner.

DAY TWELVE – FRIDAY

BREAKFAST:

Same as Day One.

LUNCH:

Fresh fruit *or* carrot juice (optional)
Energy Salad (see page 238) *or* Stuffed Pita Sandwich*

DINNER:

Fresh Vegetable Juice Cocktail (see page 241)
Curried Vegetables* and Cucumber Raita,* *or*
Broiled Fish Steaks* and Dilled Cucumbers*
Sweet Spaghetti Squash*

STUFFED PITA SANDWICH

Serves 2. *15 Min.*

Whole-wheat pita bread, which is readily available, is a great substitute for regular bread. Warm pitas briefly in oven. Do not toast, because then they are impossible to stuff. Cut off a thin strip along the top of the pita and stuff with whatever filling you prefer. Any salad you make, using fresh or steamed vegetables, or a combination of the two, can be an excellent filling for a pita sandwich. Use thicker dressings rather than drippy ones, which will soak through the bread. Eight years ago, when I was first testing new recipes, we sold pita sandwiches at our community produce store. At a time when this type of sandwich was uncommon, these were extremely popular.

Several leaves of lettuce, washed and dried
Several leaves of spinach
1 small tomato (optional) (If you are not going to eat your pita pocket immediately, you may want to omit the tomato, which has a tendency to make the pita soggy.)
1 stalk celery
½ small cucumber *or* 1 small pickling cuke
1 small carrot
½ avocado (optional)
2 cups alfalfa sprouts (optional)
1–2 tablespoons mayonnaise
½ teaspoon mustard *or* tamari
Squeeze of fresh lemon juice
Sea salt, seasoned salt, *or* salt-free seasoning (optional)
2 whole-wheat pita breads

Finely chop lettuce, spinach, tomato, celery, and cucumber, and combine in small bowl. Grate carrot and cube avocado, and add to vegetables. Add sprouts. Add mayonnaise, mustard or tamari, a squeeze of lemon, and sea salt to taste. Mix well. Stuff salad into slightly warmed pita pockets. Wrap in plastic, and store in refrigerator until you're ready to eat.

CURRIED VEGETABLES

Serves 3–4. *30 Min.*

Basic Indian cooking is actually quite easy. This is an authentic recipe I learned from a dear friend and enormously talented culinary artist from Bombay, Mrs Vasant Ullal. This is a dry curry. A wet curry variation follows the recipe.

2 teaspoons safflower oil, butter, *or* ghee (clarified butter)[4]
½ teaspoon mustard seeds (optional)
Pinch of asafetida *(hing)*[5] (optional)
1 tablespoon green chili, minced, *or* bell pepper, chopped (Use green chili if you like a hot curry.)
1 small cauliflower, cored and cut into small, fine florets
¼–½ teaspoon sea salt
1 teaspoon coriander powder
⅛ teaspoon turmeric
1 tablespoon water
1½ cups frozen petit pois
3 tablespoons coconut, finely grated
2 tablespoons fresh cilantro, finely chopped
Juice of ½ small lime

Prepare the vegetables.

In a large saucepan with lid, heat oil, butter, or ghee. Add mustard seeds, asafetida, and green chili or bell pepper. Add cauliflower. Cover and dry-steam over *very* low heat, adding sea salt, coriander, and turmeric as vegetables cook. Stir frequently. Add water if vegetables begin to stick. Cook 5–10 minutes, stirring frequently until cauliflower is tender. Add peas, mix well, and cook for 3–4 minutes longer. Stir in coconut, cilantro, and lime juice. Mix well and heat gently for a few minutes.

[4] Ghee can be purchased in Indian markets, or you can make it yourself by melting sweet butter and straining it through cheesecloth. Clarifying removes milk solids and makes butter more digestible.
[5] Indian spice used as a digestive aid in Indian cooking, available at Indian markets. Use *only* a pinch; a little goes a *long way. Hing* is another Indian name for asafetida.

Wet curry variation.
Place grated coconut in blender with ¼ teaspoon cumin, a small slice of fresh ginger, 1–2 cloves garlic, 1 teaspoon coriander, ⅛ teaspoon turmeric, and water to cover. Liquefy. Add coconut sauce at end of cooking when adding peas. Cook for 3–4 minutes. Add cilantro and lime juice.

CUCUMBER RAITA

Serves 4. *10 Min.*

This is Vasant Ullal's recipe for a cooling raita that is traditionally served with curry. Since it is made from yogurt, it makes a heavy accompaniment to any carbohydrate, such as the traditional rice or chapatis, so for this curry meal we substitute Sweet Spaghetti Squash (see page 287) to complement the Curried Vegetables and the Cucumber Raita.

- 1 small cucumber, peeled and coarsely grated
- 1½ cups plain yogurt
- 2 teaspoons safflower oil
- Pinch of asafetida *(hing)* (available at Indian markets)
- ½ teaspoon mustard seeds
- 1 tablespoon Kari Leaves *(neam)* (available at Indian markets)
- ¼ teaspoon sea salt (optional)
- 2 tablespoons fresh cilantro, chopped

In small bowl, combine cucumber with yogurt. You may want to squeeze excess water from cucumber before you add it to the yogurt. In small saucepan, heat oil. Add asafetida, mustard seeds, and curry leaves, and sizzle briefly. Pour into cucumber-yogurt mixture. Add sea salt and cilantro. Mix well.

Broiled Fish Steaks

Serves 2. *10 Min.*

2 8-ounce cuts swordfish, halibut, salmon, shark, yellowtail, *or* any thick fish steak
2 tablespoons butter, melted, *or* olive oil
Dash of Tabasco *or* cayenne pepper
¼ teaspoon sea salt, seasoned salt, *or* salt-free seasoning
Fresh ground black pepper (optional)
1 teaspoon fresh lemon juice

Preheat broiler. Wash fish steaks and pat dry. Combine all other ingredients in a small bowl. Brush both sides of fish with sauce so fish will not stick, and place in broiler, 4 inches from flame. Brush steaks frequently with sauce. Broil 3–4 minutes on each side. Be sure not to overcook fish steaks. They should be soft and moist.

Dilled Cucumbers

Serves 2–4. *15 Min.*

1 cucumber,[6] peeled, seeded, and sliced thin with carrot peeler, then julienned
½–¾ cup sour cream, depending on size of cucumber
2 tablespoons fresh lemon juice
1 teaspoon scallion, minced
2 tablespoons fresh dill, chopped, *or* 1 teaspoon dried dill
¼ teaspoon sea salt, seasoned salt, *or* salt-free seasoning

[6] If you prefer crisper cucumbers with fewer seeds, use hothouse (English) cucumbers or pickling cukes.

Combine all ingredients. Mix well. Refrigerate until ready to use. Serve as separate salad or as sauce for broiled fish.

SWEET SPAGHETTI SQUASH

Serves 6. *30 Min.*

1	medium spaghetti squash
1	tablespoon butter
4	medium carrots, finely grated
1	shallot, minced
¼	cup currants (optional)
½	cup water
1	teaspoon fresh dill (optional)
2	tablespoons pure maple syrup (optional)
1	teaspoon cinnamon
½	teaspoon cardamom
½	teaspoon sea salt (optional)
¼	teaspoon fresh ground white pepper

Cut squash in half lengthwise. Remove seeds, and place facedown in vegetable steamer, covered, over boiling water for approximately 20 minutes or until squash is tender. Cool slightly, scrape squash from shell, and set aside.

In large saucepan, melt butter. Add carrots, shallot, and currants, and sauté briefly. Add water, cover, and simmer until carrots are almost tender. Add dill, maple syrup, cinnamon, cardamom, sea salt, and pepper. Stir in squash and combine well. Simmer, covered, over low heat for 10 minutes, then remove cover and continue simmering, stirring frequently, until all water is absorbed. Serve with Curried Vegetables or in place of rice or pasta. Any leftover squash can be added to soups or stews.

MAIN-COURSE SALAD DAY

DAY THIRTEEN – SATURDAY

BREAKFAST:

Same as Day One.

LUNCH:

Continue on fruit and juice throughout the day, *or* have the Easy Fruit Salad.*

DINNER:

Fresh Vegetable Juice Cocktail (see page 241), *or*
1 papaya, *or* 1 slice of watermelon
(1–3 inches thick, cut from half melon)
California Tostada*

EASY FRUIT SALAD

Serves 2. *10 Min.*

2	apples, cored, peeled, and sliced
½	teaspoon cinnamon (optional)
2	oranges, peeled and sliced, or broken into sections
2	bananas, sliced
2	tablespoons currants
¼–½	cup fresh orange *or* apple juice (optional)

In large bowl, toss apples in cinnamon until evenly coated. Add oranges and bananas. Add currants and juice, and mix well. The currants in this salad are used to increase the concentration of fruit sugar. Since fruit is sometimes less sweet than we'd like, adding currants makes the salad more energizing. You can add currants whenever you feel a fruit salad needs some extra spark. That extra spark is *energy!*

California Tostada

45 Min.

- 1 cup fresh *or* frozen carrots, diced
- 1 cup fresh *or* frozen string beans, cut into ½-inch segments
- 1 cup fresh *or* frozen peas
- 1 cup fresh *or* frozen corn
- 6 cups iceberg lettuce, coarsely chopped
- 3 cups tortilla chips *or* 1 cup shredded Jack or Muenster cheese
- ½ cup black olives
- Fresh Tomato Salsa (see page 290)
- Great Guacamole (see page 274)
- Sour cream (optional)

Prepare the vegetables.

Place carrots and string beans in vegetable steamer, covered, over boiling water for 10 minutes. Add peas and corn, and steam for 5 minutes or until all vegetables are tender. If using fresh vegetables, you can steam carrots and string beans whole and then cut them. If using fresh corn, you can steam or boil it whole for 5 minutes and then cut from cob. If all frozen vegetables are used, the steaming time will be cut approximately in half. Combine steamed vegetables in a large bowl, and set them aside.

FRESH TOMATO SALSA:

- 3 tomatoes
- 3 tablespoons olive oil
- ½ cup red onion, minced
- 1 small green chili, minced (optional)
- 1 small red pepper, minced
- 1 small green pepper, minced
- 3 tablespoons fresh cilantro, minced
- 1 clove garlic, minced (optional)
- ½ teaspoon sea salt, seasoned salt, *or* salt-free seasoning (optional)

Prepare the salsa.

Plunge tomatoes in boiling water for a few seconds. Remove from water, and remove skins, chop into very small cubes, and set aside. Heat oil in small skillet. Add onion, and sauté until it begins to soften. Add chili and peppers, and sauté, stirring frequently, until they turn a bright color. Stir in cilantro and garlic. Allow vegetables to cool slightly, then add to tomatoes in small bowl. Add sea salt, and mix well. Set aside.

Assemble the tostada.

Mix half of vegetables with lettuce. Add half salsa to vegetable-lettuce mixture, and toss well. Stir all but ¼ cup of remaining salsa into remaining vegetables. If you are using chips, rather than cheese, place one cup tortilla chips on each of two plates. Spoon several dollops of guacamole over chips. Spoon vegetable-lettuce-salsa mixture over chips and guacamole. Spoon remaining vegetables over top. Add a dollop of guacamole and a dollop of sour cream, if desired. Spoon 2 tablespoons of remaining salsa over each tostada. Garnish with black olives and remaining chips. If you are using cheese, omit chips and sprinkle cheese on top of tostada.

NOTE: If a creamier dressing is desired, combine ¼ cup

mayonnaise with 2 tablespoons ketchup or Hain barbecue sauce, and mix into vegetable-lettuce mixture before adding it to tostada.

Place 1 peeled banana in an airtight plastic container or plastic bag in the freezer for tomorrow's Fruit Smoothie.

DAY FOURTEEN – SUNDAY

BREAKFAST:

Same as Day One, *or* Fruit Smoothie.*

LUNCH:

Fresh fruit or carrot juice (optional)
The Properly Combined Sandwich (see page 239), *or*
Vegetable Toastie,* corn chips,
and celery stalks
(Corn chips are optional. Now and then if you wish to have corn chips with a sandwich, it's all right. Two carbohydrates are an acceptable combination. If you are only looking for something crunchy to have with your sandwich, try forgoing the chips and substituting celery *or* carrot sticks.), *or*
Energy Salad (see page 238).

DINNER:

Cauliflower–Pea Cream Soup*
Tortilla Boogie,* *or* baked yam with raw butter
French Green Salad (see page 245)

Fruit Smoothie

Serves 1–2. *5 Min.*

- 1 cup fresh orange *or* apple juice
- 1 frozen *or* fresh banana
- ¼ papaya, 1 cored apple, 1 peach, *or* 1 cup strawberries, *or* 1-2 cups of any fruit you desire

Place juice, frozen or fresh banana, and fruit of your choice in blender. Liquefy.

Vegetable Toastie

Makes 1 toastie. *15 Min.*

- 1 cup mixed steamed vegetables (string beans, carrots, and cauliflower, for example)
- 1–2 tablespoons mayonnaise
- ¼ teaspoon sea salt, seasoned salt, *or* salt-free seasoning
- 1 tablespoon butter
- 2 slices whole-grain bread
- ½ cup alfalfa sprouts

Mash steamed vegetables with mayonnaise and seasoning. Butter bread. Spread vegetables on unbuttered side of one slice. Top with sprouts and second slice of bread, buttered side out. Place in toastie maker (see page 260). Heat 3 minutes each side over high flame.

Cauliflower–Pea Cream Soup

Serves 3. *35 Min.*

5 cups water
1 medium white onion, coarsely chopped
1 stalk celery, chopped
2 scallions, chopped
1 medium cauliflower, cored and chopped into 1-inch florets
1 teaspoon sea salt (optional)
1 tablespoon white miso *or* 1 vegetable bouillon
2 cups fresh or frozen peas
1 teaspoon dried dill *or 2* tablespoons fresh
1 tablespoon fresh parsley, chopped
1 teaspoon dried basil
¼ teaspoon dried sage
¼ cup fresh cilantro, chopped (optional)
2 teaspoons butter
½ teaspoon seasoned salt or salt-free seasoning (optional)

In heavy soup kettle, bring water to a boil. Add onion, celery, scallions, cauliflower, salt, and miso. Return to boil. Simmer, covered, for 10 minutes. Add peas, dill, parsley, basil, sage, and cilantro. Return to boil, cover, and simmer for an additional 10 minutes. Remove cover, and cool slightly. Purée in blender or food processor until creamy. Return to heat. Add butter, and stir as you reheat. Adjust seasonings, adding salt if desired.

NOTE: If you wish a chunky soup, you can reserve 2 cups of vegetables from the broth before puréeing and return them to soup as you reheat.

Tortilla Boogie

Serves 2–3. *25 Min.*

This is a perfect meal alternative that should be incorporated into your new eating life-style. It is fun, delicious, and extremely satisfying. We have heard from so many people that when they eat the Tortilla Boogie, they feel great the following day.

6 corn tortillas
2 tablespoons butter (optional)
An assortment of steamed vegetables, 6–7 cups whichever you desire:
Broccoli, cut into 2-inch by ½-inch lengths including floret
Cauliflower, broken into small florets
Brussels sprouts, halved or quartered
Asparagus, left whole, heavy bottom of stalk removed
Yellow squash, cut into ½-inch slices
Safflower oil *or* olive oil and lemon juice
3 cups lettuce, shredded, *or* alfalfa sprouts
1 avocado, mashed *or* sliced
Mayonnaise *or* mustard
Spike *or* salt-free seasoning

Place vegetables in steamer, covered, over boiling water for 5–7 minutes, or until tender when pierced with tip of sharp knife. Combine in large bowl. Sprinkle with a little safflower oil or olive oil and lemon juice, if desired. Heat tortillas in hot *dry* skillet, one at a time, until soft but not crisp. Place in covered casserole or between two plates with small pat of butter, if desired, on each. Place sprouts or lettuce and avocado in two small bowls. Assemble tortillas at table, with condiments and seasoning. Each person can come up with his or her own combination.

DAY FIFTEEN – MONDAY

BREAKFAST:

Same as Day One.

LUNCH:

Fresh fruit *or* carrot juice (optional)
Energy Salad (see page 238) with 1 slice buttered whole-grain toast, *or* cottage cheese, if desired

DINNER:

Fresh Vegetable Juice Cocktail, if desired (see page 241)
Carrot–Leek Bisque*
Marinated Pasta Salad*
French Green Salad (see page 245), *or* Dilled Cucumbers (see page 286)

CARROT–LEEK BISQUE

Serves 3. *30 Min.*

5	cups water
5	cups carrot slices
1	clove garlic, minced
1	small white onion, chopped
2	stalks celery, sliced
2	large leeks, sliced in rounds and soaked to remove sand
2	teaspoons dried basil
¼	teaspoon dried sage
¼	teaspoon dried thyme

1 tablespoon miso, red or white, *or* 1 vegetable bouillon
1 tablespoon sweet butter

GARNISH:

3 tablespoons sour cream (optional)
1 tablespoon chopped chives (optional)

In a soup kettle, bring water to a boil. Add remaining ingredients, except butter and garnish, in order given. Cover and bring to a boil. Simmer 20 minutes or until vegetables are soft. Remove ½ cup carrots with slotted spoon. Purée remaining soup in two increments in blender. Return to heat. Add carrots and butter. Reheat and serve. Garnish with dollop of sour cream and chopped chives, if desired. This bisque is also excellent cold.

MARINATED PASTA SALAD

Serves 3–4. *45 Min.*

2 cups broccoli florets
2 cups asparagus, sliced on the diagonal
2 cups zucchini, sliced

Prepare the vegetables.
Place broccoli, asparagus, and zucchini in vegetable steamer, covered, over boiling water for 5–7 minutes until just tender when pierced with tip of a sharp knife. Broccoli will take several minutes longer than asparagus and zucchini, so put it in steamer first. Remove vegetables from heat and reserve.

2 teaspoons olive oil
1 large shallot, minced
2 cups mushrooms, sliced
Squeeze of fresh lemon juice

Prepare the mushrooms.
In large skillet, heat oil. Add shallot and mushrooms. Sauté until mushrooms turn glossy but retain crispness, 3–4 minutes at most. Squeeze lemon juice over mushrooms, and set aside.

MARINADE:

¼ cup olive oil
1 tablespoon fresh lemon juice (optional)
½ teaspoon dried oregano *or* 2 teaspoons fresh oregano
½ teaspoon dried basil *or* 2 teaspoons fresh basil
½ teaspoon sea salt, seasoned salt, or salt-free seasoning
Fresh ground black pepper
1 clove garlic, halved or minced

Prepare the marinade.
Combine oil, lemon juice, oregano, basil, sea salt, pepper, and garlic in measuring cup. Mix well. Combine vegetables and mushrooms in large bowl. Add marinade, and toss gently. At this point vegetables can be refrigerated several hours or overnight.

½ pound De Cecco whole-wheat pasta *or* fresh vegetable fusilli
¼ cup thin red pepper strips *or* thin sun-dried tomato strips
½ cup arugula, fresh parsley, *or* fresh cilantro, chopped
¼ cup Greek olives, rinsed (optional)

Prepare the pasta.

Bring 3 quarts of water to a boil in a large kettle. Add pasta and simmer, uncovered, until just al dente, 2–3 minutes for fresh vegetable fusilli, 10–12 minutes for dried pasta. A tablespoon of olive oil may be added to water before boiling. When pasta is ready, add a cup of cold water to kettle to stop cooking. Drain immediately, and toss with marinated vegetables. Add peppers or tomatoes. Add olives and toss. Sprinkle with arugula, parsley or cilantro. Toss gently.

Freeze 2 bananas, peeled, for tomorrow's shake before going to bed.

AN ALL-FRUIT DAY FOR MAXIMUM WEIGHT LOSS!

DAY SIXTEEN – TUESDAY

You have now detoxified to the point where an All-fruit Day will be comfortable and energizing. Pace your fruit intake however you like. Have 1 or 2 large fruit meals during the day, after juice in the morning (it is easier to stay on fruit all day if you consume nothing but fresh juice in the morning), or eat smaller amounts of fruit at regular intervals throughout the day. Eat only when you are hungry. Since fruit supplies the body with the fuel it needs without a great energy expenditure, you actually may not be particularly hungry. You will unquestionably feel light and energetic.

BREAKFAST:

Fresh juice

LUNCH:

Fruit

DINNER:

Date or Strawberry Shake,* and more fruit,
1½ to 2 hours later, if desired.
You may substitute a Vegetable-fruit Platter
(see page 247) for the shake, if desired.

DATE OR STRAWBERRY SHAKE

Makes 1 large shake. *3 Min.*

- 1 cup Fresh Almond Milk (see below)
- 2 frozen bananas
- 6 pitted dates *or* 6 fresh *or* frozen strawberries

Place almond milk and fruit in blender. Blend until thick and creamy. If you like a thinner shake, use 1½ bananas.

NOTE: From now on, if you like these shakes, keep frozen bananas on hand in freezer.

These shakes are nutritious and an excellent substitute for ice cream shakes or protein drinks. Children love them.

FRESH ALMOND MILK: *10 Min.*

- ¼ cup raw almonds
- 1 cup cold water
- 2 teaspoons pure maple syrup (optional)

Nut and seed milks were used for centuries in Europe, Asia, and by the American Indians, and they are still used throughout the world as easily digestible substitutes for cow's milk. Those made from almonds or sesame seeds are excellent sources for easily assimilated calcium and they are delicious!

Blanch almonds by adding them to large skillet containing ½ inch boiling water, allowing them to sit in water as it boils for about 30 seconds. The skins will loosen noticeably. Drain and pop skins off. Place blanched almonds in blender with 1 cup cold water. Run blender at high speed for 2–3 minutes until a thick white milk has formed. If you are going to drink almond milk straight, strain it through a fine sieve. If there is a lot of pulp, you have not blended long enough. If you are going to use the milk in a shake, there is no need to strain. Add maple syrup if required.

Shakes are an ideal 'smoothing out' food after an All-fruit Day. We do not recommend having a shake on any day when you are also having cooked food.

DAY SEVENTEEN – WEDNESDAY

BREAKFAST:

Same as Day One.

LUNCH:

Fresh fruit *or* carrot juice (optional)
Energy Salad (see page 238), *or* Nuts and Cukes (see page 254)

DINNER:

Fresh Vegetable Juice Cocktail, if desired (see page 241)
Tortilla Soup*
New York Goodwich (see page 251), *or*
Perfect Corn on the Cob (see page 279)
Grandma's Coleslaw*

Tortilla Soup

Serves 5 or 6. *55 Min.*

8 cups water
1 stalk celery, chopped
1 large white onion, chopped
2 large carrots, cut into ½-inch slices
1 large carrot, finely grated
1 medium potato, peeled and cubed
2 cups cauliflower, chopped, *or* 2 cups fresh or frozen corn
4 broccoli stalks, peeled and cut into ½-inch cubes (optional)
2 cups banana squash, peeled and cut into 1-inch cubes
3 cups cabbage, sliced
1 large zucchini, sliced
1 vegetable bouillon
½ teaspoon sea salt, seasoned salt, *or* salt-free seasoning
Fresh ground black pepper
Dash of cayenne pepper
¼ teaspoon ground cumin
1 teaspoon dried oregano
4 corn tortillas
¼ cup fresh cilantro, chopped
Barbecued Onions (following)

Prepare the soup.
In a soup kettle, bring water to a boil. Add celery, onion, carrots, and potato. Cover, return to a boil, and simmer for 5 minutes. Add cauliflower, broccoli, and squash, cover, return to a boil, and simmer for 10 minutes.

BARBECUED ONIONS FOR TORTILLA SOUP:

2 tablespoons safflower oil
1 large white onion, sliced

2	tablespoons Hain *or* Robbie's barbecue sauce

Prepare the Barbecued Onions.

In large skillet, heat oil. Add onion, and sauté until it begins to soften. Add barbecue sauce, and continue sautéing, stirring frequently, until onion is thoroughly wilted. If you are having the New York Goodwich tomorrow, you can reserve ¼ cup onions, if desired.

Complete the soup.

Add cabbage and zucchini to soup. Return to boil and add bouillon, sea salt, pepper, oregano, and cumin. Stir in Barbecued Onions. Simmer for 5 minutes.

Heat tortillas in hot *dry* skillet. Cut into thick strips. Add to soup. Add cilantro. Adjust seasonings. Any leftover soup can be saved for lunch on the weekend.

GRANDMA'S COLESLAW

20 Min.

1	small head cabbage, grated *or* finely sliced
¼	cup boiling water
	Sea salt, seasoned salt, *or* salt-free seasoning
1	large carrot, peeled and finely grated
1	small green pepper, sliced very thin
	Juice of 1 small lemon
¼	cup fresh dill *or* 2 tablespoons dried dill
1–2	cups mayonnaise (Hain Saf-flower mayonnaise, if available)

Pour boiling water over cabbage. Add salt and knead well to soften cabbage. Add carrot and green pepper. Add lemon juice, dill, and mayonnaise. Mix thoroughly. Refrigerate. This coleslaw ages well in the refrigerator for days. If there is any left over, save and put it on a New York Goodwich!

DAY EIGHTEEN – THURSDAY

BREAKFAST:

Same as Day One.

LUNCH:

Fresh fruit *or* carrot juice (optional)
New York Goodwich (see page 251) *or* Energy Salad
(see page 238)

DINNER:

Fresh Vegetable Juice Cocktail, if desired
(see page 241)
Garlic Broiled Chicken,* *or* baked potato
with raw butter
Perfect Sautéed Mushrooms*
Zucchini with Basil Vinaigrette*

GARLIC BROILED CHICKEN

Serves 1–2. *25 Min.*

BASTING SAUCE:

½	teaspoon garlic, minced
1	tablespoon fresh lemon juice
1	teaspoon Dijon mustard
½	teaspoon sea salt, seasoned salt, *or* salt-free seasoning
	Fresh ground black pepper
1	whole chicken breast, halved, skinned

Combine all ingredients for basting sauce in small bowl. Brush over chicken. Broil for 10 minutes each side, 2 inches from heat, brushing frequently with sauce.

PERFECT SAUTÉED MUSHROOMS

Serves 3. *10 Min.*

- ½ pound fresh mushrooms (For maximum freshness, select only those whose caps are tightly closed around the stem.)
- 1 tablespoon butter
- Sea salt, seasoned salt, *or* salt-free seasoning (optional)
- 1 scant tablespoon fresh lemon juice

Cut ends from stems of mushrooms. Slice mushrooms lengthwise into ⅛- to ¼-inch slices. Melt butter in large skillet. Add mushrooms, tossing lightly in butter, until they just begin to soften. Add seasonings and lemon juice.

ZUCCHINI WITH BASIL VINAIGRETTE

Serves 3. *15 Min.*

- 6 small zucchini
- 1 tablespoon red onion, finely slivered
- 1 green pepper, finely julienned (optional)
- 1 red pepper, finely julienned (optional)

BASIL VINAIGRETTE:

- ¼ cup fresh basil, chopped, *or* 1 tablespoon dried basil
- 1 tablespoon fresh lemon juice

3 tablespoons olive oil
1 teaspoon Dijon mustard
¼ teaspoon sea salt, seasoned salt, *or* salt-free seasoning
Fresh ground black pepper (optional)

Cut zucchini into ¼-inch diagonals, and place in vegetable steamer, covered, over boiling water for 3 minutes or until just tender. Transfer to serving dish. Add onion and peppers, if desired. Combine vinaigrette ingredients in small bowl. Whisk and toss with vegetables, taking care not to break zucchini.

MAIN-COURSE SALAD DAY

DAY NINETEEN – FRIDAY

BREAKFAST:

Same as Day One.

LUNCH:

Continue on fruit and juice.
You may also have raw vegetables and the Vegetable-fruit Platter, if desired (see page 247).

DINNER:

½ cantaloupe, *or* ½ honeydew melon, *or* 1 whole grapefruit
Farmer's Chop Suey*

FARMER'S CHOP SUEY

Serves 2. *20 Min.*

1 small iceberg or romaine lettuce, washed, dried, and coarsely chopped
2 cups spinach, coarsely chopped
6 radishes, sliced
1 medium cucumber, peeled and sliced
1 large tomato, cubed
1 green pepper, sliced
1 small sweet red pepper, sliced (optional)
1–4 tablespoons scallions, sliced, according to taste
½ cup sour cream
1 cup creamed cottage cheese
1 teaspoon dried dill *or* 1 tablespoon fresh dill
⅛ teaspoon dried tarragon
Sea salt
Fresh ground black pepper

Combine all vegetables in large bowl. Mix together sour cream and cottage cheese in small bowl. Add dill, tarragon, sea salt, and pepper to taste. Pour over salad, and toss well. A perfect main-course salad for dairy lovers!

Freeze 1 or 2 large bananas, peeled, for tomorrow's Smoothie before going to bed.

DAY TWENTY – SATURDAY

BREAKFAST:

Same as Day One, *or* Berry Smoothie.*

LUNCH:

Fresh fruit or carrot juice (optional)
Avotillas,* *or* Energy Salad (see page 238)

DINNER:

Couscous,* and French Peas and Lettuce,* *or*
Baked Garden Vegetables*
Salade Parisienne with Asparagus (see page 270)

BERRY SMOOTHIE

3 Min.

1	cup fresh orange, apple, *or* tangerine juice
1	cup fresh or frozen berries – strawberries, raspberries, or blueberries
1 or 2	large bananas, fresh or frozen

Combine all ingredients in blender until smooth and thick. Kids love these!

NOTE: You can substitute any fruit you like for the berries.

AVOTILLAS

Serves 1. *5 Min.*

3 corn tortillas
½ avocado, cut into 6 slices
Mayonnaise *or* mustard
Spike (optional)
Alfalfa sprouts

Heat tortillas in hot *dry* skillet. Spread with mayonnaise or mustard. Place 2 slices avocado down center of each. Sprinkle with Spike. Add layer of sprouts. Roll tightly.

COUSCOUS

Serves 2–3. *15 Min.*

Couscous recipes tend to vary slightly. This one is basic, but if the recipe on your box of couscous is different, follow it. It will be correct for that particular grade of couscous.

2 cups water
1 cup couscous
2 tablespoons sweet butter
¼–½ teaspoon sea salt

Bring water to a boil. Add couscous, butter, and sea salt, and simmer, stirring continuously, for about 2 minutes or until most of water is absorbed. Remove from beat, cover, and allow to stand for 10–15 minutes.

French Peas and Lettuce

Serves 2 or 3. *20 Min.*

- 2 tablespoons sweet butter
- 1 clove garlic, halved or minced
- 3 cups fresh or frozen peas (If you are using frozen, use petit pois.)
- 1 small romaine *or* butter lettuce, coarsely chopped
- ½ teaspoon dried thyme
- ¼ cup water
- Sea salt, seasoned salt, *or* salt-free seasoning
- Additional 1 tablespoon sweet butter (optional)
- Fresh ground black pepper (optional)

Melt 2 tablespoons butter in heavy saucepan. Add garlic, and sauté 2–3 minutes to flavor butter. Remove garlic (if halved) and add peas. Sauté to coat with butter. Add lettuce, thyme, water, sea salt and pepper. Simmer, covered, over low heat for 5 minutes for frozen peas and for 10–15 minutes for fresh peas, stirring frequently to make sure peas don't burn. If water is absorbed before fresh peas are soft, add a little more. Toss with 1 tablespoon butter and pepper, if desired. Use as sauce for couscous, or combine with couscous and mix well.

Baked Garden Vegetables

Serves 4. *45 Min.*

This easy method for delicious baked vegetables will work with any assortment of vegetables except brussels sprouts, which tend to get bitter. Vegetables simply baked in butter and their own juices have a unique flavor that cannot be duplicated with other cooking methods.

1	cup carrots, cut into fine matchsticks
2	cups potatoes, peeled, quartered, and cut into ¼-inch slices *or* 1 small cauliflower, cut into ½-inch florets
1	package frozen Fordhook lima beans
2	large zucchini, quartered and cut into 1-inch cubes
2	cups cabbage or bok choy greens, coarsely chopped
¼	cup butter
3	tablespoons fresh parsley, minced (optional)
¼	teaspoon Spike or salt-free seasoning
½	teaspoon sea salt (optional)
	Fresh ground black pepper

Preheat oven to 325 degrees. Place all vegetables in heavy oven-proof casserole with lid. Dot with butter. Sprinkle with parsley, Spike, sea salt, and pepper. Cover and place in oven for 35–40 minutes or until vegetables are tender.

Toss with additional butter, if desired, and serve with salad.

Freeze 2 cups cantaloupe wedges (½ cantaloupe) in an airtight container for tomorrow's Cantaloupe Ice before going to bed.

DAY TWENTY-ONE – SUNDAY

BREAKFAST:

Fresh juice and the fruit salad of your choice, *or*
Blueberry–Cantaloupe Supreme*
and Cantaloupe Ice*

LUNCH:

Fresh fruit or carrot juice (optional)
Cuke-a-tillas (see page 266), *or* Tabouli,*
and/or Energy Salad (see page 238)

DINNER:

Fresh Vegetable Juice Cocktail, if desired
(see page 241)
Savory Cabbage Strudel,* *or* Broiled Fish Steaks
(see page 286)
Steamed Vegetables in Lemon Butter Sauce*
Dilled Cucumbers (see page 286), *or*
Grandma's Coleslaw (see page 303)

BLUEBERRY–CANTALOUPE SUPREME

10 Min.

This is a delectable summer fruit salad. Mango can be substituted for the cantaloupe. A ripe mango will be soft to pressure but not mushy. It should be very red, yellow-orange, or yellow-green. True green on a mango indicates that it is not yet ripe and will be sour. Peel the mango, and cut the fruit from the seed. Freeze summer fruits for winter enjoyment. To freeze fruits, cut them into pieces. Quarters are most convenient for peaches, nectarines, apricots, etc. Berries may be left whole. Melons should be cut into 2-inch chunks. Bananas can be frozen whole, but should be peeled first. Papayas and mangos should be peeled and cut into pieces. Fruits should be placed in airtight *containers and frozen. All frozen fruits can be turned into wonderful fruit freezes with a Champion or Oster juicer.*

½ cantaloupe, cut into bite-size cubes *or* in balls, *or* 1 mango, cut in cubes
2 Babcock peaches, peeled and sliced
1 cup blueberries
1 small banana, cut into slices (optional)

Mix all fruits together. On a hot summer day, you might want to top this salad with Cantaloupe Ice (see below) and serve it for brunch or lunch. It also makes a beautiful first course for dinner.

CANTALOUPE ICE

3 Min.

½ cantaloupe, cut into cubes and frozen

Here's another incentive to purchase a juicer, which will not only enable you to make your own fresh juices, but will also open the door to a delicious ice cream alternative: **FRESH FRUIT SOFT FREEZE!** Soft freeze is most easily prepared in a juicer. Push frozen fruit through, and out comes a marvelous frozen dessert, with no chemicals, additives, dairy products, or sugar! Any frozen fruit can be used: cantaloupe, banana, strawberries, or whatever you like. They can be used in combination or by themselves. If you don't have a juicer, soft freeze can be made in your food processor or blender.

TABOULI

Serves 4. *45 Min.*

1	cup cracked wheat (bulgur)
1½–2	cups water
½	cup fresh parsley, chopped
½	tablespoon scallions, minced
2	tablespoons fresh mint, chopped (You may substitute 2 teaspoons dried mint if fresh is not available.)
2	tablespoons olive oil
2	teaspoons fresh lemon juice
½	teaspoon sea salt, seasoned salt, or salt-free seasoning
	Fresh ground black pepper (optional)
1	small tomato, chopped (optional)

Combine cracked wheat and water, and soak until wheat is hydrated and water is absorbed, from 30–60 minutes. Add parsley, scallions, mint, olive oil, lemon juice, salt, and pepper, if desired. Mix well. Add tomato and mix gently. Serve at room temperature, or chill until ready to serve.

Savory Cabbage Strudel

Serves 3–4. *1 Hr 15 Min.*

1 tablespoon butter
4 cups cabbage, finely shredded
2 cups bok choy greens, shredded
1 tablespoon currants (optional)
1 small onion, sliced thin
2 scallions, chopped
2 tablespoons fresh dill, chopped, *or* 1 teaspoon dried dill
2 tablespoons fresh cilantro *or* parsley, chopped
½ teaspoon sea salt, seasoned salt, *or* salt-free seasoning

Prepare the filling.
Melt butter in large heavy saucepan. Add cabbage and bok choy greens, currants, onion, and scallions. Cook over medium-high heat, stirring frequently, for 3–4 minutes or until greens begin to wilt. Add dill, cilantro, and sea salt, and cook for 1 minute over high heat, stirring well to thoroughly incorporate herbs into vegetables. Set aside.

1 tablespoon butter
½ pound fresh mushrooms, sliced
1 teaspoon fresh lemon juice

Prepare the mushrooms.
In separate large skillet, melt butter. Add mushrooms, and sauté briefly over high heat, stirring frequently, until they begin to soften. Remove from heat, sprinkle with lemon juice, and add to vegetable mixture. Mix well.

4 phyllo pastry sheets (available in frozen-food section of supermarket or at food specialty shops)
2 tablespoons butter, melted
4 tablespoons dry whole-wheat bread crumbs

Assemble the strudel.
Preheat oven to 400 degrees. Strain mushroom-vegetable mixture in colander, catching liquid in small bowl. Reserve liquid to add to soup, sauces, or gravy. Lightly butter cookie sheet. Place 1 phyllo sheet on damp towel. Brush lightly with melted butter. Place second phyllo sheet on top of first. Sprinkle 2 tablespoons of bread crumbs on left-hand side of phyllo. Fold right-hand side over to encase bread crumbs, making a rectangle. Brush top lightly with melted butter. Spread ½ vegetable mixture along long edge, stopping 1 inch short of the short sides. Fold borders in to encase vegetables. Roll as you would a jelly roll. Place seam side down on buttered baking sheet. Brush roll with melted butter. Repeat for second roll. Bake until golden, about thirty minutes. Cut each into 3 or 4 sections.

STEAMED VEGETABLES IN LEMON BUTTER SAUCE

Serves 4. *20 Min.*

4–6 tender young carrots, cut into ½-inch cubes
2 medium zucchini
2 medium yellow squash
2 tablespoons butter, melted
2 teaspoons fresh lemon juice

Place carrots in vegetable steamer, covered, over boiling water for approximately 10 minutes. Add zucchini and squash, whole, and steam 5–7 minutes or until just tender. Place vegetables in serving dish. Cut squash into quarters, lengthwise, and then into ½-inch cubes. Combine butter and lemon juice in measuring cup, and pour over vegetables. Toss gently.

ALL-FRUIT DAY

DAY TWENTY-TWO – MONDAY

BREAKFAST:

Fresh fruit juice

LUNCH:

Fresh fruit juice, fruit salad of your choice, *or*
assorted pieces of fruit;
Cantaloupe Ice (see page 000), if desired

DINNER:

Fresh fruit
Date or Strawberry Shake (see page 300), if desired

The All-fruit Day is your best friend in the care, upkeep, and beautification of your body. Once you have mastered this valuable tool for weight loss and health, you are on your way to a new fitness life-style.

DAY TWENTY-THREE – TUESDAY

BREAKFAST:

Same as Day One.

LUNCH:

Fresh fruit *or* carrot juice (optional)
Nuts and Cukes (see page 254), *or* Romaine Roll-ups*

DINNER:

Fresh Vegetable Juice Cocktail, if desired (see page 241)
Bollito Misto (Steamed Vegetable Platter),* *or* Steamed Artichoke,* *and* Caesar Salad (see page 256)
Curried Corn Salad,* if desired

ROMAINE ROLL-UPS

Serves 2. *15 Min.*

This is a satisfying finger-food salad whose origin is the burrito. Crisp, slenderizing romaine lettuce leaves are used as wrappers. They are stuffed with a mixture of avocado and other vegetables.

1 large avocado
1 large tomato, coarsely chopped
1 small cucumber *or* 2 pickling cukes, peeled and chopped
1 tablespoon red onion, chopped (optional)
1–2 cups mung bean or alfalfa sprouts, or both

1	teaspoon Gulden's Spicy Brown mustard (optional)
1	tablespoon fresh lemon juice
1	head romaine lettuce, washed and dried

Slice avocado in half lengthwise. Remove seed and set aside. Scoop pulp from skin into medium-size bowl. Mash thoroughly with fork. Add tomato and cucumber to avocado. Add onion, if desired, mustard, and lemon juice. Stir in sprouts. Arrange lettuce leaves around sides of large bowl in the form of a flower. Mound avocado mixture in center. To eat, place large spoonful of avocado in center of a lettuce leaf and roll leaf burrito-style.

NOTE: If you are not using the avocado mixture immediately, place it in a container *with* the pit. This will keep it from turning brown.

BOLLITO MISTO (STEAMED VEGETABLE PLATTER)

Serves 3–4. *40 Min.*

3–4	beets
4	new potatoes, unpeeled, *or* 4 turnips, peeled
4	medium carrots *or* parsnips
3	large stalks broccoli with florets
½	medium cabbage
4	small zucchini
	OR
	Any vegetable assortment of your choice
¼	cup butter, melted, *or* Herbed Butter Sauce (see page 321)
	Squeeze of fresh lemon juice (optional)

Scrub beets and potatoes or turnips, and peel carrots. Place in vegetable steamer, covered, over boiling water for approximately 20 minutes or until tender when pierced with tip of sharp knife. Remove from heat, and peel beets, and potatoes, if desired. Set aside.

Cut thick stalks from broccoli, leaving approximately 3 inches of stem, and floret. Cut cabbage into quarters. Place broccoli, cabbage, and whole zucchini in vegetable steamer, covered, over boiling water for approximately 10 minutes or until tender. Remove from heat. Slice broccoli and zucchini lengthwise. Cut beets, potatoes, and carrots into bite-size cubes.

Arrange green vegetables in center of platter with beets, potatoes, and carrots around them. Serve with melted butter seasoned with a squeeze of lemon juice, or with Herbed Butter Sauce.

NOTE: A high-water-content steamed vegetable meal like this will speed elimination of excess weight. Make it part of your repertoire.

STEAMED ARTICHOKES

Serves 2–4. *50 Min.*

Artichokes are delicious and easy to make. Although not a heavy food, they are particularly satisfying and filling when you are craving something heavy. Make them the main part of a meal rather than the traditional first course from now on. When selecting artichokes, choose those whose petals have not opened far. The tighter and more compact the artichoke, the fresher.

4 artichokes
1 bay leaf (optional)

1 clove garlic (optional)
Several stalks celery (optional)

Cut off or trim end of artichoke stem. If desired, snip thorny tip off each leaf. Wash artichokes, taking care to shake out excess water so they will not be soggy when steamed. Place in a vegetable steamer, covered, over boiling water to which you have added bay leaf, garlic, and celery stalks. Steam for 35–45 minutes, depending on size. The artichokes are ready when one of outer leaves can easily be removed. Discard bay leaf, celery, and garlic. Serve with melted butter or Herbed Butter Sauce (see below).

HERBED BUTTER SAUCE: *7 Min.*

¼ cup butter
1 shallot, minced
1 teaspoon Dijon mustard
1 tablespoon fresh chervil *or* 1 teaspoon dried chervil
1 tablespoon fresh thyme *or* 1 teaspoon dried thyme
1 tablespoon fresh parsley, chopped
¼ teaspoon sea salt (optional)

Melt butter. Add shallot, and sauté briefly to soften. Pour butter-shallot mixture into blender. Add mustard, herbs, and salt, if desired, and blend until smooth. Serve hot, over vegetables.

CURRIED CORN SALAD

Serves 3. *20 Min.*

1	tablespoon safflower oil
½	cup red onion, finely diced
½	cup red pepper, finely diced
½	cup green pepper, finely diced
½	teaspoon curry powder
½	teaspoon dried oregano
¼	teaspoon turmeric
4	cups cooked corn (If you are using fresh corn, which is preferable in summer when it is abundant, steam corn first for 5 minutes, then cut from cob.)
½	cup pimento-stuffed green olives, sliced
½	cup mayonnaise
¾	teaspoon sea salt, seasoned salt, *or* salt-free seasoning
2	tablespoons fresh cilantro, chopped (optional)

Heat oil in large skillet. Add onion, and sauté until soft. Add red pepper and green pepper, and sauté briefly until they just begin to wilt. Add curry powder, oregano, and turmeric, and sauté briefly. Add to corn in a large bowl. Stir in olives. Add mayonnaise and sea salt, and mix well. Garnish with cilantro.

DAY TWENTY-FOUR – WEDNESDAY

BREAKFAST:

Same as Day One.

LUNCH:

Fresh fruit *or* carrot juice (optional)
Energy Salad (see page 238) *or*
New York Goodwich (see page 251)

DINNER:

Fresh Vegetable Juice Cocktail, if desired
(see page 241)
Garlic Broiled Chicken (see page 304), *or* Yam Stew*
Celeriac Salad,* *or* French Green Salad (see page 245)
Asparagus Italian Style,* *or*
Broccoli in Lemon Butter Sauce*

YAM STEW

Serves 2 as a main course. *40 Min.*

- 1 large *or* 2 small yams, peeled and quartered
- 2 crookneck squash
- 2 large zucchini
- 1 large carrot, peeled and cut into ½-inch slices
- 2 cups fresh *or* frozen lima beans *or* peas
- 2 tablespoons butter
- ½ teaspoon sea salt, seasoned salt, *or* salt-free seasoning

Place yams, squash, and zucchini in vegetable steamer covered, over boiling water for 5–7 minutes until tender. Remove squash and zucchini when tender, and allow yams to continue cooking until tender, approximately 20 minutes more. In separate steamer, steam carrots and limas for approximately 15 minutes or until tender. If using frozen limas or peas, steam carrots for 10 minutes, then add peas for another 5 minutes. If using fresh limas or peas, steam them for 20 minutes. Steam carrots for 15 minutes separately. Place carrots and limas or peas in serving dish. Cut zucchini and squash into ½-inch slices, and add to serving dish. Cut yams into 1-inch pieces, and add to serving dish. Add butter and seasoning. Toss well, and serve. The variety of flavors and textures makes this dish absolutely delightful.

CELERIAC SALAD

Serves 4. *25 Min.*

- 1 medium celeriac (celery root)
- 2 tablespoons fresh lemon juice
- ½ cup mayonnaise
- 2 teaspoons Dijon mustard

Cut celeriac into very thin slices. Cut peel from slices, then julienne each slice. Add lemon juice to 4 cups boiling water. Place celeriac in boiling water and boil 3–5 minutes or until tender-crisp. Drain well. Combine mayonnaise and mustard. Toss celeriac in the mixture. Serve at room temperature or chilled.

ASPARAGUS ITALIAN STYLE

Serves 2–4. *7 Min.*

1 pound asparagus
1 tablespoon olive oil
1 teaspoon fresh lemon juice

Break heaviest part of stalk from each asparagus spear. Wherever stalk breaks naturally is division between tender and stringy parts of vegetable. In a large saucepan, bring 2 quarts of water to a boil. Add asparagus and boil, uncovered, for 3–4 minutes until just tender-crisp. Remove asparagus from water. In serving dish, immediately toss in olive oil and lemon juice.

BROCCOLI IN LEMON BUTTER SAUCE

Serves 2–4. *10 Min.*

3–4 stalks broccoli with florets
2 tablespoons butter
2 teaspoons fresh lemon juice

Cut heavy stalks off broccoli, leaving floret and 2–3 inches of stem. Reserve stalks for Teriyaki Broccoli (see page 263), soups, or vegetable dishes. Cut each broccoli stem into individual florets. Place in steamer, covered, over boiling water 5–7 minutes. Broccoli stems should be tender when pierced with tip of sharp knife and should retain their bright green color.

In small saucepan, melt butter over low heat. Whisk in lemon juice. Pour sauce over hot broccoli.

DAY TWENTY-FIVE – THURSDAY

BREAKFAST:

Same as Day One.

LUNCH:

Fresh fruit *or* carrot juice (optional)
Stuffed Pita Sandwich (see page 282), *or*
Energy Salad (see page 238)

DINNER:

Fresh Vegetable Juice Cocktail, if desired
(see page 241)
Golden Potato Soup,* *or* Carrot-Leek Bisque
(see page 295)
Stir-fried Black Mushrooms with Zucchini and
Chinese Greens*
Dilled Cucumbers (see page 286)

GOLDEN POTATO SOUP

Serves 4. *30 Min.*

- 2 tablespoons butter
- 1 teaspoon safflower oil
- 1 clove garlic, minced
- 1 large onion, coarsely chopped
- 2 cups celery, chopped
- 5 medium russet potatoes *or* 8 White Rose potatoes, peeled and cut into 1-inch cubes
- 6–8 crookneck squash, cut into ¼-inch slices
- 1 tablespoon white miso *or* 1 vegetable bouillon

1 teaspoon dried thyme
¼ teaspoon dried tarragon
½ teaspoon dried sage
Sea salt, seasoned salt, *or* salt-free seasoning
Dash of cayenne
6–7 cups water

In heavy soup kettle, melt butter and heat oil. Add garlic, onion, and celery, and sauté until they begin to wilt. Add potatoes, squash, miso or bouillon, and seasonings. Add water to cover vegetables. Bring to a boil. Simmer, covered, for 20 minutes or until vegetables are soft. Cool slightly, and puree in increments in blender to a smooth golden cream. Reheat gently, stirring so soup doesn't stick.

STIR-FRIED BLACK MUSHROOMS WITH ZUCCHINI AND CHINESE GREENS

Serves 3–4. *45 Min.*

NOTE: *This is a basic stir-frying technique that can be used successfully with whatever vegetables you happen to have on hand. If you don't have dried mushrooms, you can substitute standard fresh mushrooms or steamed carrots. Broccoli or snow peas can be substituted for zucchini, but they should be blanched or presteamed before adding them to the wok, 1 minute of blanching for snow peas, 5 minutes of steaming for broccoli. Cabbage can be substituted for Chinese greens.*

2 cups dried black mushrooms
2 cups vegetable broth *or* soup stock
2 zucchini

6–7 scallions
1 bunch Chinese greens *or* bok choy greens (approximately 4 cups)
1 tablespoon safflower oil

Prepare the vegetables.
Soak mushrooms in vegetable broth or stock until completely hydrated, approximately 30 minutes. While mushrooms are soaking, cut zucchini and scallions into diagonal slices, and coarsely shred Chinese greens. Set aside in separate bowls. Drain mushrooms, reserving broth for sauce and final preparation. Cut heavy stems from mushrooms, and cut large ones in half. Place in bowl with zucchini.

SEASONINGS:

1 clove garlic, minced
1 teaspoon fresh ginger, minced, *or* ½ teaspoon ginger powder
Safflower oil

Prepare the seasonings.
Mince garlic and ginger. Place in small bowl, and cover with small amount of safflower oil. PLACE YOUR WOK ON HIGH HEAT AND ALLOW IT TO HEAT UNTIL YOU ARE READY TO COOK.

SAUCE:

1 cup vegetable broth from mushrooms
2 tablespoons tamari *or* thick soy sauce
1 teaspoon honey
1 tablespoon Chinese bean paste *or* tofu sauce *or* Hain barbecue sauce
2 teaspoons fresh lemon juice *or* dry sherry
½ teaspoon curry powder

Prepare the sauce.
Combine all ingredients. Mix well.

THICKENER:

1 tablespoon arrowroot *or* Japanese kuzu
2 tablespoons cold water
1 teaspoon safflower oil

Prepare the thickener.
Combine all ingredients until smooth.

Last-minute preparation.
Line up ingredients so they are easily accessible in this order: 1) oil 2) seasonings 3) scallions, zucchini and mushrooms, greens, 4) sauce, and 5) thickener.

Place oil in preheated wok. Immediately add seasonings. Immediately add scallions, and toss. Immediately add mushrooms and zucchini, continuously tossing vegetables in oil. If zucchini begins to scorch, add a few teaspoons of vegetable broth. Continue tossing until zucchini and scallions turn a bright color. Add greens. Toss continuously. Add sauce, tossing continuously until greens begin to wilt. Add thickener in a thin stream. Toss all vegetables to coat well with sauce. Turn out on platter and serve immediately.

MAIN-COURSE SALAD DAY

DAY TWENTY-SIX – FRIDAY

BREAKFAST:

Fresh fruit juice

LUNCH:

Continue on fruit and juice throughout the day.

DINNER:

1 papaya, *or* several fresh pineapple spears, *or*
1 whole grapefruit
Cantonese Seafood Salad*

CANTONESE SEAFOOD SALAD

Serves 2. *45 Min.*

- 2 cups bok choy
- 2 cups mung bean sprouts
- 2 cups snow peas
- ½ cup carrots, shredded (optional)
- 1 cup dried wood ear, cloud ear, *or* Chinese black fungus (optional),[7] presoaked for 30 minutes
- 2 teaspoons safflower oil (optional)
- 3 cups shrimp, crabmeat, *or* other seafood
- 4 cups romaine lettuce, coarsely shredded
- 2 cups spinach, coarsely shredded, *or* Chinese cabbage, finely shredded

[7]Available dried in Asian markets and fresh in finer supermarkets.

Prepare the salad.

Soak cloud ear in warm water until they swell and soften, about 30 minutes. Thinly slice bok choy. Cut through sprouts once or twice to make them bite-size. String snow peas and blanch, whole, in boiling water for 1 minute. Drain and *immediately* place under cold water or plunge into bowl of ice water. Dry and cut them into ¾-inch diagonals.

Blanch carrots for 1 minute in boiling water. Drain and immediately place under cold water or plunge into bowl of ice water.

Drain cloud ear, reserving stock for another meal. Dry them and cut into thin strips. Use raw, or sauté in oil until tender.

If using fresh shrimp, plunge them in their shells into boiling water, and boil 3–4 minutes until they turn pinkish white. Drain and run under cold water. Peel skins off, cut each shrimp in half lengthwise, and remove any waste deposits with a damp paper towel. If using frozen shrimp, steam for 3–5 minutes, undefrosted, in a vegetable steamer. Drain well. If using frozen crabmeat, defrost it, rinse, and pick out any shells. Drain well. In a large bowl, add shrimp and vegetables to greens.

CANTONESE DRESSING:

- 2 tablespoons cilantro *or* arugula, minced (optional)
- 1 tablespoon scallion, minced
- ¼ teaspoon dried ginger *or* ½ teaspoon fresh ginger, minced
- 1 teaspoon roasted sesame oil
- ½ teaspoon honey
- 2 tablespoons fresh lemon juice

2	tablespoons safflower oil
1	teaspoon Hain *or* Robbie's barbecue sauce *or* tofu sauce
1	tablespoon tamari
¼	teaspoon sea salt (optional)

Prepare the dressing.
Combine all ingredients. Mix well. Pour over salad. Toss well.

DAY TWENTY-SEVEN – SATURDAY

BREAKFAST:

Fresh juice and Fresh Applesauce*

LUNCH

Fresh fruit *or* carrot juice (optional)
Cuke-a-tillas (see page 266), *or* Avotillas (see page 309),
or Romaine Roll-ups (see page 318)

DINNER:

Fresh Vegetable Juice Cocktail, if desired (see page 241)
Harvest Soup (see page 261) *or* Old-fashioned Lentil Soup*
Honey Corn Bread,* *or* Pita Toasts*
Grandma's Coleslaw (see page 303)

Fresh Applesauce

Serves 1–2. *5 Min.*

This is a wonderful breakfast alternative, and an ideal children's food.

- ½ cup fresh apple juice *or* ½ cup water
- 2 large apples, peeled and quartered
- ½ teaspoon cinnamon or nutmeg, *or* ¼ teaspoon of each
- 1 fresh or frozen banana *or* ½ papaya *or* 2 ripe persimmons (very soft) (optional)

Place all ingredients in blender. Blend until smooth. Raw or uncooked applesauce is the only applesauce that is beneficial in our systems. Cooked applesauce is acid and does far more harm than good. Make sure this is only eaten on an empty stomach.

Old-Fashioned Lentil Soup

Serves 3 as a main course. *1 Hr 15 Min.*

- 7½ cups water
- 1 clove garlic, minced
- 1 large white onion, chopped
- 2 large carrots, coarsely chopped
- 2 stalks celery, coarsely chopped
- 1½ cups lentils
- 1 vegetable bouillon *or* 1 tablespoon red miso
- ½ teaspoon dried thyme
- 1 teaspoon dried oregano
- 1 teaspoon sweet Hungarian paprika
- ½ teaspoon Spike (optional)
- ½ teaspoon sea salt (optional)
- 1 cup fresh *or* frozen corn (optional)
- 1–2 tablespoons fresh parsley, chopped

In soup kettle, bring water to a boil. Add garlic, onion, carrots, celery, lentils, and bouillon or miso. Return to boil. Add seasonings. Mix well. Simmer, covered, over low heat for 60 minutes. If you want a creamier consistency, you can purée half the soup in blender or food processor. Return to heat and add corn, if desired. Simmer for 5 minutes. Stir in parsley.

HONEY CORN BREAD

35 Min. to 1 Hr

- 1 cup yellow cornmeal, *or* ¾ cup yellow cornmeal and ¼ cup bran
- 1 cup whole-wheat flour
- ½ teaspoon sea salt
- 1 teaspoon baking powder
- 1 teaspoon baking soda
- ¼ cup raw honey
- 1 beaten egg *or* 1 teaspoon egg replacer whipped in 1 tablespoon water
- 1⅞ cups buttermilk
- 1 teaspoon butter
- 2 cups fresh or frozen corn (optional)

Preheat oven to 375 degrees. Combine dry ingredients. Stir in liquid ingredients. Stir in corn. *Do not overmix!* Corn bread batter must be a little lumpy. Pour batter into well-buttered 8-by-8-inch pan. Bake for ½ hour without corn or 55 minutes with corn until toothpick inserted in center comes out clean. Cool slightly and cut into 2-inch squares.

NOTE: The batter for this corn bread can be prepared hours in advance and refrigerated (covered) in the baking pan until ½ hour before baking.

PITA TOASTS

Serves 4. *10 Min.*

2	whole-wheat pita breads, separated into halves
2	tablespoons butter, softened
1	small clove garlic
½	teaspoon dried thyme
½	teaspoon dried summer savory

Use garlic press to crush garlic and blend it into butter. Add herbs and mix well with fork. Spread butter on pita halves. Place under broiler for 5 minutes or until toasted.

Freeze 2–2½ bananas for tomorrow's shake before going to bed.

DAY TWENTY-EIGHT – SUNDAY

BREAKFAST:

Fresh juice, Smoothie (see pages 292 and 308) *or*
Breakfast Fruit Platter,* if desired

LUNCH:

Leftover Lentil Soup and Grandma's Coleslaw from yesterday, *or*
The Properly Combined Sandwich (see page 239), *or* Banana Shake*

DINNER:

Fresh Vegetable Juice Cocktail, if desired (see page 241)
New York Goodwich (see page 251)
Crusty Roasteds*
Leftover Grandma's Coleslaw, *or* Summer Greens with Creamy Avocado Dressing*

BREAKFAST FRUIT PLATTER

Serves 6. *15 Min.*

1 cantaloupe or Persian melon, cut into bite-size cubes
3 cups watermelon balls
4 kiwi fruit, peeled and sliced
1 large *or* 2 small papaya, peeled and sliced
2 cups seedless green grapes
6 small bunches grapes
1 large Bosc pear, peeled and cut into spears

On large round platter, combine melons, kiwi fruit, papaya, and grapes. Arrange bunches of grapes around edges of platter, alternating with pear spears.

Serve with Fruit Dip of your choice (see page 266).

BANANA SHAKE

Serves 1. *3 Min.*

- 1 cup Fresh Almond Milk (see page 300)
- 2–2½ frozen bananas (depending on size and desired thickness of shake)
- Nutmeg

In blender, combine Fresh Almond Milk, bananas, and nutmeg to taste. Blend until creamy.

CRUSTY ROASTEDS

Serves 2–3. *35 Min.*

These are a delicious alternative to french fries, and you'll love them if potatoes are one of your addictions. You'll find them to be a really terrific 'non-fried potato treat.' Although they are wonderful, overeating them will halt your progress. Take it easy! Don't stuff yourself. Look at this as a treat and not a binge so you can enjoy these roasteds in your new life-style repertoire.

- 5 new potatoes
- 1–2 tablespoons butter, melted
- Dash of Spike, Herbit, *or* seasoning of your choice

Place potatoes in vegetable steamer, covered, over boiling water for 20 minutes or until they test tender when pierced with tip of sharp knife. Do not allow them to get too soft. Cool potatoes and cut into ¼-inch slices. Place on cookie sheet, and brush evenly with butter. Sprinkle with seasoning, and place as close as possible to heat of broiler until crusty and golden, approximately 10 minutes. It is not necessary to turn them.

Summer Greens with Creamy Avocado Dressing

Serves 2. *15 Min.*

An assortment of lettuce – several leaves each of butter, romaine, salad bowl, and red leaf
2 cups spinach
1 cup arugula (optional)
1 small cucumber, peeled and sliced, *or* 2 pickling cukes, peeled and sliced
2 cups sprouts – alfalfa, buckwheat, *or* sunflower
½ cup olives (optional) *or* 1 cup enoki mushrooms

Prepare the salad.
Wash and thoroughly dry lettuce and break into bite-size pieces, discarding center rib. Break spinach into bite-size pieces. Combine lettuce and spinach in large bowl. Add arugula, if desired, cucumber, and sprouts.

CREAMY AVOCADO DRESSING: *Makes 2 cups*

1 avocado
1 small clove garlic, minced
¼ cup water
2 teaspoons olive oil

2	tablespoons sour cream
1	tablespoon fresh dill *or* 1 teaspoon dried dill
½	teaspoon honey
½	teaspoon sea salt, seasoned salt, *or* salt-free seasoning
2	tablespoons fresh lemon juice

Prepare the dressing.

Cut avocado in half. Peel, remove pit, and cut into large cubes. Place all ingredients in food processor or blender. Process until creamy and smooth. Use as dressing for Summer Greens, as dip for raw or steamed vegetables, or as topping on sandwiches.

Assemble the salad.

Pour ½ cup of dressing over greens. Toss well. Add a few tablespoons additional dressing, if desired. Add olives or enoki mushrooms, if desired. Toss lightly.

In Conclusion

A tremendous effort has gone into perfecting this system over the last fifteen years. Obviously it is not a 'hit-and-run,' on-again off-again approach. Its purpose is to put you in harmony with your physiological needs and your natural body cycles and to show you how to eat to optimize both. With this information you will always have control over your energy and your weight.

If you are not yet the weight you wish to be, be assured that you will arrive there if you continue to eat properly combined, high-water-content meals and nothing but fruit in the morning. Just proceed! You are still in the process of acquiring your **LIFETIME ENERGY LIFE-STYLE**. If you continue to do what has been outlined, the weight will continue to come off, and it will be gone for good as you become more energetic and healthy.

If you wish to accelerate your progress, skip around in the program and emphasize the high-energy days that call for fruit all day with a high-water-content Main-Course Salad or a New York Goodwich in the evening. These are the days when you will experience maximum weight loss. Two exceedingly important guidelines should be kept in mind: First, that concentrated foods, proteins and carbohydrates, should be properly combined and not account for more than 30 per cent of your food intake for any one day; second, fruit is your absolute best friend in the upkeep and care of your body. Correctly consumed and eaten in sufficient quantities, fruit will insure that you will never have a weight problem again.

The most important feature of this approach to eating is the fact that it's a LIFE-STYLE, not a dogmatic set of rules that must be adhered to by rote. This affords you the opportunity to participate to the extent that it appeals to you personally. You can pick and choose what areas are attractive to you. If there are certain aspects that appeal to your common sense, that you feel can be utilized without pressure, let that be your STARTING POINT! By keeping your destination in mind and doing *something,* no matter how little, every day, there will be sufficient momentum to keep the ball rolling. You *will* ultimately reach your destination. And you will reach it a happier, healthier person. The key is DIRECTION, not speed.

We're thrilled that we have been able to assist you in losing weight, and we are doubly thrilled that we've been able to help you improve the length and quality of your life.

These pages contain a lifelong system. You can always refer to them for help. Even if you 'waver from the path' and gain unwanted weight or experience a state of low energy, years from now you will always have the tools to turn the situation around and regain your vitality. You can always depend on the natural laws of life, and this system is built on those laws.

You have taken responsibility for your body. Thinner, looking and feeling better every day, you can enjoy every minute of your newfound vibrant energy.

You have put in the effort to obtain it, and you most assuredly deserve it!

HEALTH AND VITALITY, WITH ALL THEIR BENEFITS, ARE NOTHING LESS THAN YOUR BIRTHRIGHT!

MAY HEALTH ALWAYS BE YOUR GOAL AND YOUR REWARD!

* * *

Bibliography

Abramowski, O.L.M., M.D. *Fruitarian Healing System*. Natal, South Africa: Essence of Health, 1976.

—— *Fruitarian Diet and Physical Rejuvenation*. Wethersfield, Connecticut: Omangod Press, 1973.

Accraido, Marcia M. *Light Eating for Survival*. Wethersfield, Connecticut: Omangod Press, 1978.

Agres, Ted. *Your Food, Your Health*. Chicago: Inter-Direction Press, 1972.

Airola, Paavo. 'Meat for B_{12}?' *Nutrition Health Review* (Summer 1983): 13.

Allen, Hannah. *The Happy Truth About Protein*. Austin, Texas: Life Science, 1976.

—— 'Lesson #33, Why We Should Not Eat Animal Products in Any Form.' In *The Life Science Health System*, by T. C. Fry. Austin, Texas: Life Science, 1984.

Altman, Nathaniel. *Eating for Life*. Wheaton, Illinois: Theosophical Publishers, 1974.

Ames, Bruce N. 'Dietary Carcinogens and Anti-Carcinogens.' *Science*, 23 September 1983: 1256.

Armstrong, J. W. *The Water of Life*. Devon, England: Health Science Press, 1978.

Bach, Edward. *Heal Thyself*. London: Daniel, 1946.

Ballentine, Martha. *Himalayan Mountain Cookery*. Honesdale, Pennsylvania: Himalayan International Institute, 1978.

Barr, Stringfellow, and Stella Standard. *The Kitchen Garden Book*. New York: Viking Press, 1956.

Bauman, Edward, et al. *The Holistic Health Handbook*. California: And/Or Press, 1978.

Bealle, Morris A. *The Drug Story.* Spanish Fork, Utah: The Hornet's Nest, 1949.

—— *The New Drug Story.* Washington, D.C.: Columbia Publishing Co., 1958.

Beiler, Henry G. *Food Is Your Best Medicine.* New York: Random House, 1965.

Benerjee, D. K., and J. B. Chatterjea. 'Vitamin B Content of Some Articles of Indian Diet and Effect of Cooking on It.' *British Journal of Nutrition* 94 (1968): 289.

Benson, Herbert. *Beyond the Relaxation Response.* New York: Times Books, 1984.

Benton, Mike. 'Lesson #30, Sugars and Other Sweeteners May Be Worse Than Bad.' In *The Life Science Health System,* by T. C. Fry. Austin, Texas: Life Science, 1984.

—— 'Lesson #34, The Harmfulness of Beverages in the Diet.' In *The Life Science Health System,* by T. C. Fry. Austin, Texas: Life Science, 1984.

Bernard, Raymond W. *Eat Your Way to Better Health,* Vol. I & II. Clarksburg, West Virginia: Saucerian, 1974.

—— *Rejuvenation Through Dietetic Sex Control.* Natal, South Africa: Essence of Health, 1967.

Bernard, Theos. *Heaven Lies Within Us.* Natal, South Africa: Essence of Health, 1947.

Bianchi, Paul, and Russel Hilf. *Protein Metabolism and Biological Function.* New Brunswick, New Jersey: Rutgers University Press, 1970.

Bigwood, E. J. *Protein and Amino Acid Functions.* New York: Pergamon Press, 1972.

Bircher-Benner, M. *Eating Your Way to Health.* Baltimore, Maryland: Penguin, 1973.

Biser, Samuel. 'The Truth About Milk.' *The Healthview Newsletter* 14 (Spring 1978): 1–5.

Bodwell, C. E. *Evaluation of Protein for Humans.* Westport, Connecticut: The Air Publishing Company, 1977.

Bond, Harry C., M.D. *Natural Food Cookbook.* North Hollywood, California: Wilshire Book Co., 1974.

Bricklin, Mark. *The Practical Encyclopedia of Natural Healing.* Emmaus, Pennsylvania: Rodale Press, 1976.

Brooks, Karen. *The Complete Vegetarian Cookbook.* New York: Pocket Books, 1976.

Brown, Henry. *Protein Nutrition.* Springfield, Illinois: Charles C. Thomas Publishers, 1974.

Burton, Alec, Ph.D. 'Milk.' *Hygienic Review,* July 1974.
Callela, John. *Cooking Naturally.* Berkeley, California: And/Or Press, 1978.
Cancer Facts and Figures. American Cancer Society, 1983.
'Can Fruit Help You Lose Weight?' *Bergen Record,* 20 October 1983.
Carmichael, Dan. 'Milk Surplus Continues to Grow as Price Climbs Even Higher.' *St. Petersburg Times,* 3 June 1982.
Carque, Otto. *Vital Facts About Food.* New Canaan, Connecticut: Keats, 1975.
Carrington, Hereward, Ph.D. *The History of Natural Hygiene.* Mokelhumne Hill, California: Health Research, 1964.
Carter, Mary Ellen, and William McGarey. *Edgar Cayce on Healing.* New York: Warner, 1972.
Cheraskin, Emanuel, M.D., W. Ringsdorf, M.D., and J. W. Clark. *Diet and Disease.* Emmaus, Pennsylvania: Rodale Press, 1968.
Cinque, Ralph. 'Losing Weight Hygienically.' *Health Reporter* 8 (1983): 5.
Claire, Rosine. *French Gourmet Vegetarian Cookbook.* Millbrae, California: Celestial Arts, 1975.
Colgate, Doris. *The Barefoot Gourmet.* New York: Offshore Sailing School, 1982.
Cornelius, Martin P., III. *'Til Death Do Us Part.* Los Angeles, California: Healer, 1981.
Cousins, Norman. *Anatomy of an Illness.* New York: Bantam Books, 1979.
D'Adamo, Janus, M.D. *One Man's Food.* New York: Richard Marek, 1980.
Dauphin, Lise, N.D. *Recettes Naturistes.* Montreal, Canada: Editions Du Jour, 1969.
Dash, Bhagwan. *Ayervedic Treatment for Common Diseases.* New Delhi: Delhi Diary, 1979.
De Vries, Herbert A. *Vigor Regained.* Englewood Cliffs, New Jersey: Prentice-Hall, 1974.
Diamond, Marilyn. *The Common Sense Guide to a New Way of Eating.* Santa Monica, California: Golden Glow Publishers, 1979.
'Diet and Stress in Vascular Disease.' *Journal of the American Medical Association* 176 (1961): 134.
Dossey, Larry, M.D. *Space, Time and Medicine.* Boulder, Colorado: Shambala, 1982.
Dosti, Rose. 'Nutrition Needs Greater for Pregnant Teen-agers, Over 30s.' *Los Angeles Times,* 31 May 1984.

Ehret, Arnold. *Mucusless Diet Healthing System.* New York: Benedict Lust, 1976.
Esser, William L. *Dictionary of Man's Foods.* Chicago: Natural Hygiene Press, 1972.
Farb, Peter, and George Armelagos. *The Anthropology of Eating.* Boston: Houghton Mifflin Co., 1980.
Farnsworth, Steve. 'Plan to Cut Milk Surplus Isn't Working.' *Los Angeles Times,* 5 March 1984.
Fathman, George, and Doris Fathman. *Live Foods.* Beaumont, California: Ehret Literature Publishing, 1973.
Finkel, Maurice. *Fresh Hope in Cancer.* Devon, England: Health Science Press, 1978.
Ford, Marjorie Winn, Susan Hillyard, and Mary E Koock. *Deaf Smith Country Cookbook.* New York: Collier Books, 1974.
Friedlander, Barbara. *Earth, Water, Fire, Air.* New York: Collier Books, 1972.
Fry, T. C. *The Cruel Hoax Called Herpes.* Austin, Texas: Life Science, 1983.
—— *The Curse of Cooking.* Austin, Texas: Life Science, 1975.
—— *The Great Water Controversy.* Austin, Texas: Life Science, 1974.
—— *High Energy Methods, Lessons 1-7.* Austin, Texas: Life Science, 1983.
—— *The Life Science Health System, Lessons* I-III. Austin, Texas: Life Science, 1983.
—— *The Myth of Medicine.* Austin, Texas: Life Science, 1974.
—— *The Revelation of Health.* Austin, Texas: Life Science, 1981.
—— *Super Food for Super Health.* Austin, Texas: Life Science, 1976.
—— *Superior Foods, Diet Principles and Practices for Perfect Health.* Austin, Texas: Life Science, 1974.
Garrison, Omar V. *The Dictocrats.* Chicago: Books for Today, 1970.
Gewanter, Vera. *A Passion for Vegetables.* New York: Viking Press, 1980.
Glaser, Ronald. *The Body Is the Hero.* New York: Random House, 1976.
Gore, Rick. 'The Awesome Worlds Within a Cell.' *National Geographic* 3 (1976): 355.
Gould, George M., and Walter L. Pyle. *Anomalies and Curiosities of Medicine.* New York: The Julian Press, 1956. Originally copyright 1896.
Gray, Henry, M.D. *Gray's Anatomy.* New York: Bounty Books, 1977.

Griffin, LaDean. *Is Any Sick Among You.* Provo, Utah: Bi World, 1974.
Gross, Joy. *The Vegetarian Child.* New York: Lyle Stuart, 1983.
—— *Positive Power People.* Glendora, California: Royal CBS Publications, 1981.
Guyton, Arthur C. *Guidance Textbook of Medical Physiology.* Philadelphia: Saunders Publishing Co., 1981.
—— *Physiology of the Body.* Philadelphia: W. B. Saunders, 1981.
'Heart Facts.' American Heart Association, 1984.
Heritage, Ford. *Composition and Facts About Foods.* Mokelhumne Hill, California: Health Research, 1971.
Hewitt, Jean. *The New York Times Natural Foods Cookbook.* New York: Avon, 1972.
—— *The New York Times NEW Natural Foods Cookbook.* New York: Times Books, 1982.
Hightower, Jim. *Eat Your Heart Out.* New York: Random House, 1976.
Holmberg, Osterholm, et al. 'Drug Resistant Salmonella from Animals Fed Antimicrobials.' *New England Journal of Medicine* 311 (1984): 617.
Hopkins, S. F, F.P.S. *Principal Drugs.* London: Faber & Faber, 1969.
Hotema, Hilton. *Perfect Health.* Natal, South Africa: Essence of Health, no date in book.
Hovannessian, A. T. *Raw Eating.* Tehran: Arshavir, 1967.
Howell, W. H., M.D. *The Human Machine.* Ontario, Canada: Provoker Press, 1969.
Hunter, Beatrice T. *Consumer Beware: Your Food and What's Been Done to It.* New York: Simon & Schuster, 1972.
Hur, Robin A. *Food Reform – Our Desperate Need.* Herr-Heidelberg, 1975.
Hurd, Frank J., D.C., and Rosalie Hurd, B.S. *Ten Talents.* Chisholm, Minnesota: Dr. & Mrs. Frank J. Hurd, 1968.
Illich, Ivan. *Medical Nemesis.* New York: Bantam, 1976.
Jensen, Bernard, D.C. *The Science of Iridology.* Escondido, California: Jensen's Nutritional & Health Products, 1952.
Khalsa, Siri V.K. *Conscious Cookery.* Los Angeles: Siri Ved Kaur Khalsa, 1978.
Klinger, Rafe. 'Amazing 142-year-old Man Is Actually Growing Younger, Say Stunned Doctors.' *Weekly World News,* 7 October 1980.
Krok, Morris. *Amazing New Health System.* Natal, South Africa: Essence of Health, 1976.

—— *Formula for Long Life*. Natal, South Africa: Essence of Health, 1977.
—— *Fruit, the Food and Medicine for Man*. Natal, South Africa: Essence of Health, 1967.
—— *Golden Path to Rejuvenation*. Natal, South Africa: Essence of Health, 1974.
—— *Health, Diet and Living on Air*. Natal, South Africa: Essence of Health, 1964.
—— *Health Truths Eternal*. Natal, South Africa: Essence of Health, 1964.
Kulvinskas, Victoras. *Survival into the 21st Century*. Wethersfield, Connecticut: Omangod Press, 1975.
Kushi, Michio. *Macrobiotics*. Tokyo, Japan: Japan Publications, 1977.
—— *Oriental Diagnosis*. London, England: Red Moon, 1978.
Laurel, Alicia B. *Living on the Earth*. New York: Vintage, 1971.
Leaf, Alexander, M.D. 'Every Day Is a Gift When You Are Over 100.' *National Geographic* 1 (1973): 93–119.
Leonardo, Blanche. *Cancer and Other Diseases from Meat*. Santa Monica, California: Leaves of Healing, 1979.
Levy, Stuart. 'Playing Antibiotic Pool.' *New England Journal of Medicine* 311 (1984): 663.
Lewis, David L. 'Henry Ford and the Wayside Inn.' *Early American Life* 5 (1978): 5.
Long, James W., M.D. *The Essential Guide to Prescription Drugs*. New York: Harper & Row, 1980.
Longwood, William. *Poisons in Your Food*. New York: Pyramid, 1969.
Luce, Gay Gaer, Ph.D. *Body Time: Physiological Rhythms*. New York: Pantheon, 1971.
Mallos, Tess. *Complete Middle East Cookbook*. New York: McGraw-Hill, 1982.
Mayer, Jean, and Jeanne Goldberg. 'More Cancer Causes Studied.' *Los Angeles Times*, 9 September 1982.
McBean, Eleanor. *The Poisoned Needle*. Mokelhumne Hill, California: Health Research, 1974.
McCarter, Robert, Ph.D., and Elizabeth McCarter, Ph.D. 'A Statement on Vitamins,' 'Vitamins and Cures,' 'Other Unnecessary Supplements.' *Health Reporter* 11 (1984): 10, 24,
Mendelsohn, Robert S., M.D. *Confessions of a Medical Heretic*. New York: Warner Books, 1980.

——*How to Raise a Healthy Child in Spite of Your Doctor.* Chicago: Contemporary Books, 1984.
Montagna, Joseph F. *People's Desk References,* Vol. I & II. Lake Oswego, Oregon: Quest for Truth Publications, 1980.
Moore-Ede, Martin C. *The Clocks That Time Us.* Boston, Massachusetts: Harvard University Press, 1982.
Morash, Marian. *The Victory Garden Cookbook.* New York: Knopf, 1982.
Muktananda, Swami. *Play of Consciousness.* New York: S.Y.D.A. Foundation-Om Namah Shivaya, 1978.
Munro, H. N., et al. *Mammalian Protein Metabolism.* New York: Academic Press, 1970.
Nance, John. *The Gentle Tasaday.* New York: Harcourt Brace Jovanovich, 1975.
Nasset, E. S. 'Amino Acid Homeostasis in the Gut Lumen and Its Nutritional Significance.' *World Review of Nutrition and Dietetics* 14 (1972): 134–153.
Nelson, Harry. 'Patients Want Doctor to Talk More.' *Los Angeles Times,* 30 November 1978.
Newman, Laura, M.D. *Make Your Juicer Your Drugstore.* Simi Valley, California: Benedict Lust, 1972.
Nolfi, Cristine, M.D. *My Experiences with Living Food.* Ontario, Canada: Provoker Press, 1969.
Norman, N. Philip, M.D. 'Food Combinations: An Original Scheme of Eating Based upon the Newer Knowledge of Nutrition and Digestion.' *Journal of the Medical Society of New Jersey* 12 (1924): 375.
Null, Gary. *Food Combining Handbook.* New York: Jove, 1981.
Okitani, A., et al. 'Heat Induced Changes in Free Amino Acids on Manufactured Heat Pulp and Pastes from Tomatoes.' *The Journal of Food Science* 48 (1983): 1366-1367.
'Opening Executive Gyms to All Trims Waists, Health Costs.' *Los Angeles Times,* 19 April 1981.
Ouseley, S.G.J. *The Power of the Rays.* London: L.N. Fowler & Co., 1972.
Overend, William. 'Looking for Cancer Clues in Survey.' *Los Angeles Times,* 24 September 1983.
Page, Melvin, and H. L. Abrams. *Your Body Is Your Best Doctor.* New Canaan, Connecticut: Keats, 1972.
Parham, Barbara. *What's Wrong with Eating Meat?* Denver, Colorado: Ananda Marga Publications, 1979.

Parish, Peter, M.D. *The Doctor's and Patient's Handbook of Medicines and Drugs.* New York: Knopf, 1978.

Pasley, Salley. *The Tao of Cooking.* Berkeley, California: Ten Speed Press, 1982.

Pasta. Alexandria, Virginia: Time-Life Books, 1982.

Pavlov, Ivan P. *The Work of the Digestive Glands.* London: Griffin, 1902.

Pottenger, F. M., Jr. 'The Effect of Heated, Processed Foods and Vitamin D Milk on the Dental Facial Structure of Experimental Animals.' *American Journal of Orthodontics and Oral Surgery:* Aug. 1946.

Randolph, Theron G., M.D., and Ralph W. Moss, Ph.D. *An Alternative Approach to Allergies.* New York: Lippincott & Crowell, 1979.

Rensberger, Boyce. 'Research Yields Surprises About Early Human Diets.' *The New York Times,* 15 May 1979.

Reuben, David, M.D. *Everything You Always Wanted to Know About Nutrition.* New York: Avon, 1979.

Richter, Vera. *Cook-Less Book.* Ontario, Canada: Provoker Press, 1971.

Rivers, Francis. 'The Passing Parade.' *Nutrition Health Review,* Winter 1981: 19.

'Rolling Along.' *Los Angeles Times,* 18 December 1980.

Rombauer, Irma S., and Marion R. Becker. *Joy of Cooking.* New York: Signet, 1973.

Ruehl, Franklin R. 'Eating Fruit Can Cut Your Heart Attack Risk.' *The National Enquirer,* 11 January, 1983.

Sahni, Julie. *Classic Indian Cooking.* New York: William Morrow & Co., 1980.

Sandler, Sandra and Bruce. *Home Bakebook of Natural Breads and Cookies.* Harrisburg, Pennsylvania: Stackpole, 1972.

San Francisco Muktananda Center. *So What's Cooking?* Oakland, California: S.Y.D.A. Foundation, 1979.

Saunders, David S. *An Introduction to Biological Rhythms.* New York: Wiley, 1977.

Scharffenberg, John A., M.D. *Problems with Meat.* Santa Barbara, California: Woodridge Press, 1979.

Schell, Orville. *Modern Meat.* New York: Random House, 1984.

Select Committee on Nutrition and Human Needs, U.S. Senate. *Dietary Goals for the United States.* Washington, D.C.: U.S. Government Printing Office, 1977.

Shelton, Herbert M., Ph.D. *Exercise.* Chicago: Natural Hygiene Press, 1971.
—— *Fasting Can Save Your Life.* Chicago: Natural Hygiene Press, 1964.
—— *Food Combining Made Easy.* San Antonio, Texas: Dr Shelton's Health School, 1951.
—— *Getting Well.* Mokelhumne Hill, California: Health Research.
—— *Health for All.* Mokelhumne Hill, California: Health Research.
—— *Human Beauty, Its Culture and Hygiene.* San Antonio, Texas: Dr Shelton's Health School, 1968.
—— *Human Life, Its Philosophy and Laws.* Mokelhumne Hill, California: Health Research, 1979.
—— 'The Digestion of Milk.' *Hygienic Review:* August 1969.
—— *The Hygienic Care of Children.* Bridgeport, Connecticut: Natural Hygiene Press, 1981.
—— *The Hygienic System,* Vol. I, II, & III. San Antonio, Texas: Dr Shelton's Health School, 1934.
—— *Natural Hygiene, Man's Pristine Way of Life.* San Antonio, Texas: Dr Shelton's Health School, 1968.
—— *Principles of Natural Hygiene.* San Antonio, Texas: Dr Shelton's Health School, 1964.
—— *Rubies in the Sand.* San Antonio, Texas: Dr Shelton's Health School, 1961.
—— *Superior Nutrition.* San Antonio, Texas: Dr Shelton's Health School, 1951.
Silverman, Harold M., (Pharm. D.) and Gilbert I. Simon, D.Sc. *The Pill Book.* New York: Bantam, 1979.
Singer, Peter, and Jim Mason. *Animal Factories.* Bridgeport, Connecticut: Natural Hygiene Press, 1980.
Snodgrass, Beth. *Overcoming Asthma.* Austin, Texas: Life Science, 1968.
—— *Overcoming Asthma.* Yorktown, Texas: Life Science, 1980.
Spencer, R. P. *The Intestinal Tract.* Springfield, Illinois: Charles Thomas Publishers, 1960.
Stern, Edward L. *Prescription Drugs and Their Side Effects.* New York: Grosset & Dunlap, 1978.
Su-Huei, Huang. *Chinese Appetizers and Garnishes.* Taipei, Taiwan: Huang Su-Huei, 1983.
Sunset International. *Vegetarian Cookbook.* Menlo Park, California: Lane Publishing, 1983.
Tannahill, Reay. *Food in History.* New York: Stein & Day, 1981.

Thomas, Anna. *The Vegetarian Epicure,* Books I & II. New York: Knopf, 1972.
Tilden, John H., M.D. *Toxemia Explained.* Denver: Health Research, 1926.
Time-Life. *Vegetables.* Alexandria, Virginia: Time-Life Books, 1979.
Tobe, John H. *Hunza: Adventures in a Land of Paradise.* Ontario, Canada: Provoker Press, 1971.
Trall, Russell T., M.D. *The Hygienic System.* Battle Creek, Michigan: The Office of the Health Reformer, 1872.
Verrett, Jacqueline, and Jean Carper. *Eating May Be Hazardous to Your Health.* New York: Simon & Schuster, 1974.
'Vitamins of the B Complex.' *United States Department of Agriculture Yearbook.* Washington, D.C.: 1959.
'Vitamin Megadoses Can Be Harmful.' *Los Angeles Times,* 20 December 1983.
Waerland, Are. *Health Is Your Birthright.* Bern, Switzerland: Humata Publishers, *Circa* 1945.
Waerland, Ebba. *Cancer, a Disease of Civilization.* Ontario, Canada: Provoker Press, 1980.
Waldholz, Michael, and Richard Koening. 'New Ulcer Drug Near Approval, Setting Up a Big Fight with SmithKline's Top Seller.' *The Wall Street Journal,* 12 November 1982.
Walker, N. W., D.Sc. *Become Younger.* Phoenix, Arizona: Norwalk Press, 1949.
—— *Diet and Salad Suggestions.* Phoenix, Arizona: Norwalk Press, 1971.
—— *Fresh Vegetables and Fruit Juices.* Phoenix, Arizona: Norwalk Press, 1978.
—— *Natural Weight Control.* Phoenix, Arizona: O'Sullivan Woodside & Co., 1981.
—— *Vibrant Health.* Phoenix, Arizona: O'Sullivan Woodside & Co., 1972.
—— *Water Can Undermine Your Health.* Phoenix, Arizona: O'Sullivan Woodside & Co., 1974.
'What Americans Don't Eat – Some Surprises.' *Grocers Journal of California,* September 1982: 87.
'Whole Milk Linked with Cancer.' *Nutrition Health Review,* Spring 1983.
Wigmore, Ann. *Be Your Own Doctor.* Boston: Hippocrates Health Institute, 1973.
Winter, Ruth. *Beware of the Food You Eat.* New York: Signet, 1971.

Index

Abkhazians of Russia, 70
Acid
build up of, 56, 79, 80, 96–98, 162–63
from dairy products, 148
hyperacidity, 93
Additives, chemical, 133, 143–44, 177
Aerobic exercise, 151–55
Airola, Paavo, 136n.
Ak Mak-Ararat Bakeries, Division of Soojian, Inc., 215, 216
Albert Lucas products, 220
Alcoholic beverages, 100, 167, 177
Alcott, Dr. William, 42
Allen, Hannah, 140, 147n.
Allergies, 140, 145, 149
Almond Milk
Banana Shake, 337
Date or Strawberry Shake, 300
Fresh, 300
Alta Dena Dairies, 218
American Academy of Pediatrics, 20
American Cancer Society, 115
American College of Health Science, 41, 43, 52, 119, 128, 187
American College of Surgeons, 93
American Heart Association, 241
American Natural Hygiene Society, 43–4, 51
American Physiological Society, 42
Ames, Dr. Bruce, 165
Amino acids, 95, 98, 123–31, 137
pool of, 127–29
see also Protein
Anabolism, 55
Ananda Products, 214, 216, 220
Anatomy of an Illness (Cousins), 157
Anomalies and Curiosities of Medicine (Gould and Pyle), 128n.
Antacids, 79
Antibiotics, 134, 144
Anxiety, 112
Appetite, loss of, 135
Apple(s), 190, 202
Applesauce, Fresh, 333
dried, 208
Easy Fruit Salad, 288–89
Apple juice
Berry Smoothie, 308
Fruit Smoothie, 292
Appropriation cycle, 52, 72, 75, 108
Apricots, 202
dried, 208
Arrowhead Mills, Inc., 215, 216, 219
Arrowroot, 220
Arthritis, 120, 140, 145
Artichokes, 208
Steamed, 320–1
Arugula for French Green Salad, 245–46

Asparagus, 174, 208
Curried Chicken Salad, 258–59
Italian Style, 325
Marinated Pasta Salad, 296–98
Salade Parisienne with, 270
Aspinal, John, 123n.
Assimilation cycle, 53, 56, 72, 81, 95, 108–9, 155
Asthma, 140, 149
Athletes, 135
Avocado, 207, 240
Avotillas, 309
Dressing, Creamy, 338–39
Great Guacamole, 274
Properly Combined Sandwich, The, 239–41
Romaine Roll-ups, 318–19
Vegetable-Fruit Platter, 247
Avotillas, 309
Award-Winning Potato-Lovers' Salad, 271–73
Aware Inn, 219

Baked Garden Vegetables, 310–11
Banana(s), 101, 129, 191, 194, 202
Berry Smoothie, 307, 308
dried, 208
Easy Fruit Salad, 288–89
Fruit Smoothie, 291, 292
Shake, 337
Strawberry–Kiwi Salad, 265
Bárány, Robert, 126
Barbara's Chips, 214, 216
Barbecued Onions, 252, 302–3
Barbecue sauce, 220
Barley, 214
Basil
Carrots, Sweet, 269
Vinaigrette, Zucchini with, 305–6
Beans, 83n., 129, 174, 209
see also individual types of beans
Beef, *see* Meat
Beets, 208
Beliefs and your body's condition, 157–60
Benerjee, D. K., 136n.
Benson, Dr. Herbert, 20n., 157
Benton, Mike, 119
Bergen Record, 94
Berries, 202
Smoothie, 308
see also individual types of berries
Beth Israel Hospital, Boston, 157
Beverages, 100, 161–65, 167, 195–97
alcoholic, 100, 167, 177
juices, *see* Juices
shakes, *see* Shakes
Beyond the Relaxation Response (Benson), 157
Bianchi, C. Paul, 128*n.*
Bigwood, E. J., 131n.
Bircher-Benner, M., 174n.
Birth defects, 162, 177
Biser, Samuel, 145n.
Bisque, Carrot–Leek, 295–96
Bladder cancer, 93
Bloating, 57, 97, 112
Blood, 45, 151
Bloomfield, Dr. Harold, 20n.
Blueberry–Cantaloupe Supreme, 312–13
Blue Ribbon Split Pea Soup, 276
Bodwell, E. J., 131n.
Body cycles, *see* Natural body cycles
Bok choy, 208
Cantonese Seafood Salad, 330–32
Crusty Butter-Crumb Vegetables, 274–75
Savory Cabbage Strudel, 315–16
Stir-Fried Black Mushrooms with Zucchini and Chinese Greens, 327–29
Bollito Misto (Steamed Vegetable Platter), 319–20
Boston, Massachusetts, 20, 42
Bouillon, 221
Brain, 46, 172
Bread(s), 213
Cauliflower Toastie, 260–61
Crusty Butter-Crumb Vegetables, 274–75
Pita
Stuffed Sandwich, 282–83

Toasts, 335
sandwich, 239
see also Sandwiches
Shepherd's Pie, 267–69
shopping list, 213
Vegetable Toastie, 292
Breakfast, 29, 190–94, 237
guidelines, 194
skipping, 53, 102–4
Breakfast Fruit Platter, 336
Breast cancer, 93
Breast-feeding, 184–85
Brenner, Dr. Paul, 20n.
Broccoli, 208
in Lemon Butter Sauce, 325
Marinated Pasta Salad, 296–98
New York Goodwich, 251–53
Potato-Lovers' Salad, Award-Winning, 271–73
Teriyaki, 263–4
Broiled Fish Steaks, 286
Broth, 221
Brown, Dr. Henry, 128n.
Brussels sprouts, 129, 208
Bulgur, *see* Cracked wheat
Burton, Alec, 140
Butter(s), 148, 218, 230
Crumb Vegetables, Crusty, 274–75
Hot, Corn Tortillas, 262–63
Nut, Dip, 250
Sauce
Herbed, 321
Lemon Butter, Broccoli in, 325
Lemon, Steamed Vegetables in, 316–17
Buttermilk for Honey Corn Bread, 334

Cabbage, 129, 174, 208
Coleslaw
Grandma's, 303
Tangy Green, 264
Crusty Butter-Crumb Vegetables, 274–75
Curried, 257
Harvest Soup, 261–62
Split Pea Soup, Blue Ribbon, 276
Strudel, Savory, 315–16
Caesar Salad, 256
Caffeine, 161–62, 164, 165, 177
Cafix, 223
Calcium, 147–48, 174, 175, 176, 185, 230
California, 20n.
California Medical Association, 20
California Tostada, 289–91
Calories, counting, 28, 105–6
Cancer, 50, 63, 70, 115
diet and prevention of, 115, 140
foods linked to, 120, 162, 164–65
protein consumption and, 93
Cancer and Other Diseases from Meat Consumption (Leonardo), 93n.
Cannibalism, 137–38
Cantaloupe
Breakfast Fruit Platter, 336
Ice, 311, 313–14
Supreme, Blueberry–, 312–13
Cantonese Dressing, 331–32
Cantonese Seafood Salad, 330–32
Capello's Gourmet Food Products, 220
Carbohydrates, 130, 135, 172
see also Starches
Carbonic acid, 164
Carnivores, 131–33
Carrot(s), 129, 208
California Tostada, 289–91
Crusty Butter-Crumb Vegetables, 274–75
Fresh Vegetable Juice Cocktail, 241
Harvest Soup, 261–62
Hash Browns, 263
–Leek Bisque, 295–96
Steamed Vegetables in Lemon Butter Sauce, 316–17
Stew for Two, 255
Sweet Basil, 269
Yam Stew, 323–24
Case for Health, A (Diamond), 196n.
Casein, 143, 147, 174
Cason, Dr. Arthur, 80

Castelli, Dr. William, 94, 115
Catabolism, 55
Cauliflower, 129, 174, 208
  Crusty Butter-Crumb Vegetables, 274–75
  Curried Vegetables, 283–85
  Harvest Soup, 261–62
  New York Goodwich, 251–53
  –Pea Cream Soup, 293
  Soup, Perfect Creamy, 242–43
  Toastie, 260–61
Cedarlane, 214, 216
Celery, 208
  Fresh Vegetable Juice Cocktail, 241
Celery root (celeriac), 208
  Salad, 324
Celestial Seasonings, 163, 223
Cells, 127, 157–58
  composition of, 46–7
  reproduction, 46
Cellulite, 98
Cereals, 213–17
Cesar Cardini Foods, 219
Champion juicer, 197, 313
Chard, 208
Chatterjea, J. B., 136n.
Cheese, 145–46, 218
  California Tostada, 289–91
Chemical-free foods, 200–1, 230
Chemicals in meats, 134, 137, 144
Cherimoya, 204
Cherries, 202
Chicken
  Easy Roast, 244
  Garlic Broiled, 304–5
  Salad, Curried, 258–59
  see also Meat
Children, 149, 165, 192–94, 229
Chips, 214–15
Chocolate, 165–67
Chop Suey, Farmer's, 307
Chowder, Country Corn, 250–51
  see also Soup(s)
Cinque, Dr. Ralph, 32, 175, 175n.
Circadian rhythms, 52
Cleansing, *see* Detoxification; Elimination cycle
Coffee, 100, 161–63, 196
  decaffeinated, 162
  substitutes, 223
  Colds, 140, 193
Colitis, 113
Columbia University, Institute of Human Nutrition, 168, 176
Combining foods, principle of properly, 74–90
  the digestive process and, 74–83
  increased energy resulting from, 75, 84, 86, 87–89
  weight loss resulting from, 84, 88–90
  when to eat fruit, 95–96, 97–98, 101–2, 103–5, 190–94, 230, 249, 281, 317
Common Sense Guide to a New Way of Eating, The, (Diamond), 188n.
Concentrated foods, 61, 62, 64–66, 71, 145
  digesting, 77, 81, 82–84
  at salad bars, 226–27
Condiments, *see* Seasonings and condiments
Cooking, 99, 131, 229–31
Corn, 129, 209
  Bread, Honey, 334–35
  California Tostada, 289–91
  Chowder, Country, 250–51
  on the Cob, Perfect, 279
  Salad, Curried, 322
Cornell University, 164
Cornell University Medical Center, 85
Cornish hens, *see* Meat
Cottage Cheese for Farmer's Chop Suey, 307
Country Corn Chowder, 250–51
Couscous, 214, 309
Cousins, Dr. Norman, 20n., 157
Cracked wheat (bulgur), 214
  Tabouli, 314
Crackers, 215

Cravings, 68, 187
Creamy Avocado Dressing, 338–39
Creamy Dressing, 272
Croutons, Garlic, 256–57
Crusty Butter-Crumb Vegetables, 274–75
Crusty Roasteds, 337–38
Cucumbers, 129, 207
  Cuke-A-Tillas, 266
  Dilled, 286–87
  Energy Salad, 238
  Nuts and, 254
  Properly Combined Sandwich, The, 239–41
  Raita, 285
  Vegetable-fruit Platter, 247
Currants, 208
Curried Cabbage, 257
Curried Chicken Salad, 258–59
Curried Corn Salad, 322
Curried Mayonnaise Dressing, 259
Curried Vegetables, 283–85
Cyborski, Cathy Kapica, 135n.

Dacopa Foods, 223
Daikon, 209
Dairy Council of California, 176
Dairy products, 139–50, 217–18, 230
  shopping list, 218
  see also individual dairy products
Dandelion greens, 209
Date(s), 101, 147, 191, 203
  Shake, 300
Degenerative diseases, 32, 49–50, 63, 70, 115, 140
  see also individual diseases, e.g. Arthritis; Cancer; Heart diseases
Dehydration, 112, 135
Depression, 184, 186
De Schryver, Adrien, 123n.
Detoxification, 63–73, 76–77, 187, 188
  discomfort from, 110–15
  fruit consumption and, 94–96, 107–8
  theory of, 110–18
Detoxification Workshops, 188–89
Deviating from the program, 32, 116–17
Diabetes, 162
Diamond, Harvey (author), 27–179, 184, 187, 196
Diamond, Marilyn (author), 59, 181–342
Diarrhea, 112, 135
Diet and Salad Suggestions (Walker), 147n., 174n.
'Diet and Stress in Vascular Disease,' 135n.
Diet for a Small Planet (Lappé), 25
Dietary Goals for the United States, 49
Diets
  fad, 31, 33–4
  ineffectiveness of, 35–9
Digestive system, 45–6, 76, 79
  dairy products, digestion of, 143, 174
  energy required for digestion, 76–77, 81, 95–96, 99, 102–3, 121
  meat-eating and suitability of human, 130–33
  properly combined foods to aid, 77–90
Dijon Dressing, 281
Dilled Cucumbers, 286–87
Dinner, 30
  four-week sample menus and recipes, 235–339
  substituting a main-course salad for, 225–26, 229
Dip
  Fruit, 266
  Great Guacamole, 274
  Nut Butter, 250
Disease, 32, 50, 63, 71
  defining, 18–19
  degenerative, *see* Degenerative diseases
  diet and, 115, 120
DNA, 47, 166

Dr. Bronner's All-One-God-Faith
Inc., 214, 217, 220
Dolomite, 176
Dosti, Rose, 175n.
Dressings, *see* Salad Dressing(s)
'Drug Resistant Salmonella from
Animals Fed Antimicrobials,'
144n
Drugs, 111, 177
Ducellier, Armand, 186
Dulse, 147

Ear infections, 140, 149, 193
Early American Life (Lewis), 87
Easy Fruit Salad, 288–89
Easy Roast Chicken, 244
Eating Your Way to Health (Bircher-
Berner), 174n.
Eden Foods, 210, 215, 219, 220, 221
Edward and Sons, 215, 217
Eggplant, 129, 209
Eggs, 137
Einstein, Albert, 129
Elimination cycle, 53–54, 56, 58, 88,
107–8, 155, 190, 192–3
high-water-content food, 63–64,
72–73
theory of detoxification, 110–18
see also Detoxification
Ellis, Dr. William A., 145
El Molino Mills, 215, 216
Endive, Belgian, 209
Energy, 102
balance, 13, 18, 19, 31, 32–33, 42
dairy product consumption as
drain on, 143
to digest food, 76–77, 80, 95,
102–3, 121
Energy Ladder, 198–99
increased, 75–76, 86, 88, 89, 114
Energy Salad, 238
Erythorbic acid, 164
Evaluation of Proteins for Humans
(Bodwell), 131n.
*Everything You Always Wanted to
Know About Nutrition*
(Reuben), 49

Exercise, 135, 151–56
Eyes, circles under the, 98

Fad diets, 31, 33–34
Farmer's Chop Suey, 307
Fat (dietary), 115, 130, 148, 218
Fatigue, 112, 145
Fatty acids, 95, 98
Feces during detoxification period,
112
Fennel, 209
Fermentation, 79, 80, 84, 107, 165,
167
Fiber, 130, 166
Figs, 147, 174, 203, 208
Fingernails, 148–49
Finn Crisp-Wasa Bread-Shaffer
Clarke, Inc., 215, 216
Fish
shopping list, 218
Steaks, Broiled, 286
FIT FOR LIFE program
breakfast, *see* Breakfast
guidelines, 194
dairy products, 139–50
dinner, *see* Dinner
energy increases from, *see* Energy
the Energy Ladder, 198–99
exercise as part of, 151–56
four-week example of, 235–339
guidelines
breakfast, 194
life-style, 229–31
lunch, *see* Lunch
the main-course salad, 224–28
menus, 235–339
natural body cycles, 52–4
Natural Hygiene, 40–51
permanent results of, 28, 30–1
portion size, 189, 190–91, 229
positive beliefs and, 157–60
principle of correct fruit
consumption, 91–109, 172,
191, 230
principle of high-water-content
food, 60–73, 105

principle of proper food combining, 30, 74–90, 145
protein, 119–38
questions and answers about, 161–78
recipes, 235–339
shopping list for, 200–23
substitutions, 225–26, 229–30
theory of detoxification, 110–18
theory of metabolic imbalance, 55–59
what it isn't, 28
when to eat, 30, 98–102
fruit, 95, 96, 101, 103, 190, 230, 249, 281, 317
Flatulence, 79, 81, 83n., 113
Flesh food, *see* Meat
Flours and meal, 215
Food and Drug Administration, 134
Food combining, *see* Combining foods, principle of properly
Food for Life, 213, 216
Food Reform – Our Desperate Need (Hur), 136n., 174n.
Ford, Henry, 87
Formula, 185
Foundation for Nutritional Research, 165
Four-food-group myth, 84–85
Fourteenth Annual Nutrition Conference, 176
Framingham Study on Heart Disease, 94
French Dressing, 270
French Green Salad, 245–46
French Peas and Lettuce, 310
Fresh air, 155–56, 178
Fresh Applesauce, 333
Fresh Tomato Salsa, 290
Frieda of California, 204
Fructose, 94, 95, 172
Fruit, 61, 66, 95–96, 166, 168, 174
Breakfast, Platter, 336
breakfast suggestions, 190–94
calcium content of, 147–48
canned, 29
Dip, 266
dried, 101, 191, 208
exotic, 204–6
fresh, 29, 99, 100, 229–31
as high-water-content food, 62, 66, 93
hypoglycemics and, 171–73
juices, *see* Juices, fruit
principle of correct fruit consumption, 91–109, 172, 230
the digestive process, 95, 100
instinctive cravings, 92
when to eat fruit, 95–96, 97–98, 101–2, 103–5, 190, 230, 249, 281, 317
Salad, Easy, 288–89
at salad bars, 227
shopping list, 201–8
Smoothie, 292
vegetable, 207, 247
see also individual types of fruit
Fry, T. C, 43, 52, 120, 121n., 128, 131n., 136n.

Gaer-Luce, Gay, 52
Galileo, 85–86
Garden of Eatin', 213, 214, 216
Garlic, 209, 230
Broiled Chicken, 304–5
Croutons, 256–57
Herb Dressing, 248–49
String Beans, 244–45
Gas, 79, 81, 83n., 112, 113
Gayelord Hauser Products, 221, 222
Glucose, 95, 98, 172–73
Glucose Tolerance Test, 173
Glycerine, 95
Golden Eagle products, 219
Golden Potato Soup, 326–27
Goodwich, New York, 251–53
Gould, George M., 138n.
Gout, 120
Gove, Dr. Mary, 42
Graber Co., C. C., 220
Graham, Dr. Sylvester, 42

Grains
  shopping list, 213–17
  see also individual types of grains
Grandma's Coleslaw, 303
Grapefruit, 203
Grapes, 203
  Breakfast Fruit Platter, 336
Gravy, Mushroom Cream, 268–69
Great Guacamole, 274
Greece, 42
Green beans, 209
  California Tostada, 289–91
  Garlic String Beans, 244
  Steak-Lovers' Salad, 280
Grocers Journal of California, 140
Gross, Joy, 32, 126*n.*
Guava, 205
Guidance Textbook of Medical Physiology (Guyton), 121n..
Guidelines
  breakfast, 194
  life-style, 229–31
Guyton, Arthur C., 121n., 126n., 128

Habits, changing your eating, 116
Hain products, 213, 219, 220
Hair
  balding, 98
  graying, 98
  loss, 148
Harris, David, 20n.
Harris poll, Louis, 37
Harvard Medical School, 94, 115
Harvard University, 157
Harvest Soup, 261–62
Hav-A-Corn – Hav-A Natural Foods, 215, 217
Hay fever, 140
Health Reporter, 32, 169n.
Health Valley Natural Foods, 215, 216, 219
Heart, 45, 151, 154
Heartburn, 79, 81, 82, 96
Heart diseases, 50, 63, 64, 93–94, 115, 120, 135, 140, 145
'Heat Induced Changes in Free Amino Acids on Manufactured Heated Pulps and Pastes from Tomatoes,' 131n.
Herb(s)
  Dressing, Garlic, 248–49
  shopping list, 221–22
Herbed Butter Sauce, 321
High blood pressure, 120, 162, 170
High-water-content food, 81, 93, 105, 192, 227
  principle of, 60–73
  see also Fruit; Vegetable(s)
Hilf, Russell, 128n.
Hindus, 129
Hippocrates, 42
Holistic approach to health, 20
Holmberg, Dr., 144
Hollywood Health Foods, 219, 220
Homeostasis, 18, 21
Honey Corn Bread, 333–34
Hot Buttered Corn Tortillas, 262–63
How to Raise a Healthy Child in Spite of Your Doctor (Mendelsohn), 184–85, 185n.
Hufnagel, Dr. Vicki G., 176
Human body, Natural Hygiene and a healthy, 44–9
Hunzas, 129
Hunzukuts of Pakistan, 70
Hur, Robin A., 136n., 174n.
Hygiene, *see* Natural Hygiene
Hygienic Care of Children, The (Shelton), 147n., 174, 174n.
Hygienic System, The (Trall), 42
Hygienic System, Vol. II, The (Shelton), 80
Hypertension, *see* High blood pressure
Hypoglycemia, 171–73

Ice cream, 146
Ices, Cantaloupe, 313–14
Indigestion, 79, 81, 96
Inglefinger, Dr. Franz, 20n.
Ingrasci, Dr. Rick, 20n.
Insulin, 162
Integrative medicine, 20–21

International Congress on Obesity, 94
International Society for Research on Civilization and Environment, 137n.
International Society for Research on Nutrition and Vital Statistics, 137
Intestinal Tract, The (Spencer), 136n.
Intestines, 80, 132
'Intrinsic factor,' 136

Jennings, Dr. Isaac, 42
Jerusalem artichokes, 209
Jicama, 209
Johns Hopkins University, 92
  School of Medicine, 85
Journal of the American Medical Association, 74, 135, 135n.
Joy, Dr. Brugh, 20n.
Juicer, 190, 195, 197, 313–14
Juices
  fruit, 29
    breakfast suggestions, 190–94
    fresh, 99–100, 195–97
    when to consume, 95–96, 97–98, 101–2, 103–5
  vegetable, 30, 100, 195–97
    Cocktail, Fresh Vegetable, 241–2

Kale, 129, 209
Kasha, 214
Keeler, Richard O., 140
Kelp, 147
Kettle Chips – N. S. Khalsa, 215, 217
Kidneys, 137, 162, 167, 169, 170
Kiwi, 205
  Breakfast Fruit Platter, 336
  Strawberry–, Salad, 265
Kleeman, Dr. Charles, 20n.
Kling, Joyce M., 174n.
Kulvinskas, Viktoras, 93n., 120, 126n., 136n., 140
Kuzu, 220

Labels, reading, 200
Lactase, 143, 174
Lappé, Frances Moore, 125
Law of minimum, 169
Lawrene, Kay S., 13–16
Leaf, Alexander Dr., 70
Learning disabilities, 193
Lee, Dr. Royal, 165
Leek(s), 209
  Carrot–, Bisque, 295–96
Legumes, 217
Lemon Butter Sauce, 316–17, 325
Lentil Soup, Old-Fashioned, 333–34
Leonard, George, 20n.
Leonardo, Blanche, 93n., 120
'Lesson #8, Proteins in the Diet,' 121n., 131n.
'Lesson #33, Why We Should Not Eat Animal Products in Any Form,' 147n.
'Lesson #55, Prenatal Care for Better Infant and Maternal Health and Less Painful Childbirth', 174n., 175n.
Lettuce, 174, 209
  California Tostada, 289–91
  French Peas and, 310
  Properly Combined Sandwich, The, 239–41
  Romaine Roll-Ups, 318–19
  see also Salad(s)
Leukemia, 93
Levy, Dr. Stuart, 144n.
Lewis, David L., 87
Life Science Health System, The (Fry), 126n., 131n.
Life span, 18, 32, 70
Lifestream Natural Foods, Ltd., 213, 216
Life-style, 28–32, 106–7, 154, 340–42
  guidelines, 229–31
Light Dressing, 239
Lima beans, 209
  Yam Stew, 323–24
List of foods you ate in one day, 60, 71
Live Food Products, 220

Liver, 127, 132, 137, 167, 169
cancer, 93
Lo Mein with Shredded Vegetables, Stir-Fried, 277–78
Loquat, 205
Los Angeles Times, 70, 140, 141, 168
Lumholtz, Dr. Carl, 137
Lunch, 29
four-week sample menus and recipes, 235–339
substitution of fresh fruit for, 230
Lungs, 46
Lychee, 205
Lymph system, 127

McBean, Eleanor, 164
McCarter, Drs Robert and Elizabeth, 169n.
McCay, Dr. Clive, 164
Macrobiotics, 99
Main-course salad, 224–28, 246
as dinner substitute, 225–26, 229
substituting one, for another, 225–26
Malic acid, 164
Mammalian Protein Metabolism (Munro *et al*), 128n.
Mammals, eating patterns of, 66–72
Mango, 205, 312
dried, 208
'Man Who Lives with Gorillas, The,' 123n.
Marinated Pasta Salad, 296–98
Mayo, William J., 93
Mayo Clinic, 93
Mayonnaise, 220
Dressing, Curried, 259
Meal, *see* Flour and meal
Meat, 122–25, 185, 280
carnivore versus human physiology, 130–33
chemicals given to animals, 133, 134, 137, 144
hints to minimize negative effects of eating, 133–35
shopping list, 218
when to eat fruit after eating, 101
see also Chicken; Fish
'Meat for B_{12},' 136n.
Mediterranean Rice Salad, 247–48
Melons, 190, 192, 194, 203
Cantaloupe Ice, 311, 313–14
Breakfast Fruit Platter, 336
Supreme, Blueberry–, 312–13
Mendelsohn, Dr. Robert S., 184–85
Menstrual cycle, 230
Menus, four-week sample, 235–339
Metabolic imbalance, theory of, 55–59
Mi-Del Honey Grahams – Health Foods, Inc., 215, 216
Migraine headaches, 140, 145
Milk, 19, 21, 100, 140–50, 184–85, 196
Almond, Fresh, 300
digesting, 146, 174
see also Dairy products
Minerals, 62, 71, 94, 98, 175
supplements, 167–70, 176
Miso, 220
Modern Products, Inc., 221
Mother Earth Chips – Enterprises, Inc., 215, 217
Mucus, 112–13, 143, 144–45, 193
Munro, H. N., 128n.
Muscular system, 46
Mushrooms, 209–10
Black, with Zucchini and Chinese Greens, Stir-Fried, 327–29
Cream Gravy, 268–69
Marinated Pasta Salad, 296–98
Perfect Sautéed, 305
Mustard, 220
Dijon Dressing, 281
Mustard greens, 210

Nasset, E. S., 128
National Academy of Science, 20
National Cancer Institute, 115
National Geographic, 70
National Institutes of Health, 241
Natural and Kosher Foods, Inc., 214, 216

Natural body cycles, 52–4, 107–9, 188
Natural Hygiene, 40–51, 55, 59, 184, 187
as basis for FIT FOR LIFE program, 50
definition of, 44–5
history of, 40–3
proponents of, 42–3
see also FIT FOR LIFE program
Natural laws, 31, 32, 44
Natural Weight Control (Walker), 69
Nausea, 112
Nectarines, 203
Nephritis, 170
New England Journal of Medicine, 144
New York Goodwich, 251–53
New York Times, 92
Noodles, Lo Mein, with Shredded Vegetables, Stir-Fried, 277–78
Norman, Dr. Philip, 75
Nutrition, 15, 18
well-being and, 49–51
'Nutritional Needs Greater for Pregnant Teenagers, Over 30s,' 175n.
Nutrition Health Review, 134, 136n.
Nuts, 129, 147, 149, 174, 211–12, 230
butters, 213
Dip, 250
and Cukes, 254
shopping list, 211–12

Oasis Health Breads, Inc., 213, 216
Obesity, 50, 54, 70, 78, 84, 98, 145
of mammals, 66–67
theory of metabolic imbalance, 55–59
Oils shopping list, 219
Okitani, A., 131n.
Okra, 129
Old-Fashioned Lentil Soup, 333–34
Old Monk products, 219
Olives, 220
Onions, 210, 230
Barbecued, for New York Goodwich, 252
for Tortilla Soup, 302–3
Orange(s), 190, 203
Easy Fruit Salad, 288–89
Strawberry–Kiwi Salad, 265
Orange juice, 174
Berry Smoothie, 308
Fruit Smoothie, 292
Osteoporosis, 120
Osterholm, Dr., 144
Oster juicer, 197, 313
Overeating
avoiding, 191, 232–34
in pregnancy, 176–77
reasons for, 233

Panasonic juicer, 197
Pancreatic cancer, 162
Papaya, 206
Breakfast Fruit Platter, 336
dried, 208
Parham, Barbara, 120
Parsley Patch, Inc., 221
Parsnips, 210
'Passion to Protect,' 123n.
Pasta(s), 215
Salad, Marinated, 296–98
Pavlov, Ivan, 74
Peaches, 203
Blueberry–Cantaloupe Supreme, 312–13
dried, 208
Peanuts, 129, 213
Pears, 204
dried, 208
Breakfast Fruit Platter, 336
Peas, 129, 210
California Tostada, 289–91
Cream Soup, Cauliflower–, 293
Curried Vegetables, 283–85
French, and Lettuce, 310
Snow, *see* Snow peas
Split Pea Soup, Blue Ribbon, 276
Yam Stew, 323–24
Penicillin, 133, 144

Peppers, 207
Perfect Corn on the Cob, 279
Perfect Creamy Cauliflower Soup, 242–43
Perfect Sautéed Mushrooms, 305
Persimmon, 206
Perspiration, 132
pH balance, 163, 164
Phosphoric acid, 164
Physiology of the Body (Guyton), 126n., 128
Pickles, 220
Pineapple, 190, 204
  dried, 208
Pion, Dr. Ron, 20n.
Pionier, 223
Pita
  Sandwich, Stuffed, 282–83
  Toasts, 335
Pizza, 146
'Playing Antibiotic Pool,' 144n.
Plums, 204
Poisoned Needle, The (McBean), 164
Pomegranate, 206
Pork, *see* Meat
Positive outlook, 157–60
Positive Power People (Gross), 32
Potato(es), 129, 210
  Boats, 243–44
  Carrot Hash Browns, 263
  Country Corn Chowder, 250–51
  Crusty Roasteds, 337–38
  Harvest Soup, 261–62
  -Lovers' Salad, Award-Winning, 271–73
  Shepherd's Pie, 267–69
  Soup, Golden, 326–27
  Stew for Two, 255
Pottenger, F. M., 140
Poultry, *see* Meat
Pregnancy, FIT FOR LIFE program during, 173–78
Presco Food Products, 221
President's Council on Physical Fitness, 140
Pribram, Dr. Karl, 20n.
Principle of correct fruit consumption, 91–109, 173–74
  digestive process, 95, 100
  instinctive cravings, 92
  when to eat fruit, 95–96, 97–98, 101–2, 103–5, 190, 230, 249, 281, 317
Principle of high-water-content food, 60–73, 107
Principle of proper food combining, 74–90, 145
  digestive process and, 74–82
  increased energy resulting from, 75–76, 86, 88, 89, 114
  weight loss resulting from, 84, 88
Processed foods, 57, 147, 177
Properly Combined Sandwich, The, 239–41
Protein, 119–38, 211–12
  animal, 122–38
  assimilation of, 120
  combining proteins and, 83–84
  combining starches and, 80–82, 83–84, 87, 226–27
  overconsumption of, 93, 121, 125
  plant, 124–29, 135
  requirements, 121–22
  see also Amino acids
  Protein and Amino Acid Functions (Bigwood), 131n.
Protein Metabolism and Biological Function (Bianchi and Hilf), 128n.
Protein Nutrition (Brown), 128n.
'Protein Supplements and Body Building Programs,' 135n.
Prunes, 147, 208
Ptyalin, 131
Pure & Simple, Inc., 220, 221
Putrefaction, 79, 80, 84, 107, 137
Pyle, Dr. Walter L., 138n.

Questions and answers about FIT FOR LIFE program, 161–78

Radishes, 210
Raisins, 208

Rebounding, 152
Renin, 143, 173
Respiratory ailments, 140
Restaurants, eating in, 88–89
Reuben, Dr. David, 49
Rice, 214
  Salad, Mediterranean, 247–48
Rice Cakes – Arden Organics, Inc., 215
Richmond, Dr. Julius, 20n.
Ringing in the ears, 162
Robbie's Natural Products, 220
Rodin, Judith, 94
Romaine Roll-ups, 318–19
Rombouts, 223
Rutabagas, 210

Salad(s)
  Blueberry–Cantaloupe Supreme, 312–13
  Caesar, 256
  Cantonese Seafood, 330–32
  Celeriac, 324
  Curried Chicken, 258–59
  Curried Corn, 322
  Energy, 238
  Farmer's Chop Suey, 307
  French Green, 245–46
  Fruit
    Breakfast, Platter, 336
    Easy Salad, 288–89
  the main-course, 224–28, 229, 246
  Marinated Pasta, 296–98
  Mediterranean Rice, 247–48
  Parisienne with Asparagus, 270
  Potato-Lovers', Award-Winning, 271–73
  Spinach–Sprout, 253
  Steak-Lovers', 280–81
  Strawberry–Kiwi, 265
  Stuffed Pita Sandwich, 282–83
  Summer Greens with Creamy Avocado Dressing, 338–39
Salad bars, 226–28
Salad dressing(s), 219, 227, 230
  Cantonese, 331–32
  Creamy, 272
  Creamy Avocado, 338–39
  Curried Mayonnaise, 259
  Dijon, 281
  French, 270
  Garlic Herb, 248–49
  Light, 239
  see also Sauce(s)
Salade Parisienne with Asparagus, 270
Saliva, 100, 131
Salsa, Fresh Tomato, 290
Salt, 170, 177, 220–21
  seasoned, 221
  substitutes, 220–21
Sandwich(es)
  New York Goodwich, 251–53
  Properly Combined, The, 239–41
  Stuffed Pita, 282–83
Sapote, 206
Saturated fat, 131
Sauce(s)
  Herbed Butter, 321
  Lemon Butter, 316–17, 325
  see also Salad dressing(s)
Savory Cabbage Strudel, 315–16
Scharffenberg, John A., 120
Schell, Orville, 120
Seafood Salad, Cantonese, 330–32
Sea salt, 170
Seasonings and condiments, 220–22
Sea vegetables, 210
Seeds, 147, 149, 174, 212–13
  butters, 213
  shopping list, 212–13
  Seelect Inc., 223
  Semmelweis, Ignaz, 19
Sesame seeds, 129, 147, 174, 212
Shake(s)
  Banana, 337
  Berry Smoothie, 308
  Date or Strawberry, 300
  Fruit Smoothie, 292
Shallots, 211
Shelton, Dr. Herbert M., 43, 74, 80, 96, 120, 140, 147n., 149, 174, 174n.
Shelton Farms Poultry, 218

Shepherd's Pie, 267–69
Shopping list, 200–23
Sidhwa, Dr. K. R., 43
Skeletal system, 46
Skin, 45–6, 98, 148
Smith, Dr. Gerard, 85
Smoking, 177
Snap beans, 211
Snodgrass, Beth, 149
Snow peas, 211
  Cantonese Seafood Salad, 330–32
Soda, 100, 164–65, 196
Soken Trading, Inc., 215, 216, 221
Soup(s)
  Carrot–Leek Bisque, 295–96
  Cauliflower–Pea Cream, 293
  Creamy Cauliflower, Perfect, 242–3
  Chowder, Country Corn, 250–51
  Golden Potato, 326–27
  Harvest, 261–62
  leftover, 230
  Lentil, Old-Fashioned, 333–34
  Split Pea, Blue Ribbon, 276
  Tortilla, 302–3
Source, The, 219
Sour cream, 218
  Dilled Cucumbers, 286–87
  Farmer's Chop Suey, 307
Sovex Natural Foods, 216
Soy Sauce, 221
Spencer, R. P., 136n.
Spices shopping list, 222
Spinach, 211
  –Sprout Salad, 253
  see also Salad(s)
Sprouts, 211
  Cantonese Seafood Salad, 330–32
  Energy Salad, 238
  Properly Combined Sandwich, The, 239
  Romaine Roll-ups, 318–19
  Spinach–, Salad, 253
Squash, 129, 211
  Crusty Butter-Crumb Vegetabtes, 274–75
  Harvest Soup, 261–62
  Potato Boats, 233–34
  Spaghetti, Sweet, 287
  Steamed Vegetables in Lemon Butter Sauce, 316–17
  Yam Stew, 323–24
  zucchini, *see* Zucchini
Starches, 131
  combining protein and, 80–82, 83, 87, 226–27
  combining starches and, 84
  see also Carbohydrates
Steak-Lovers' Salad, 280–81
Steamed Artichokes, 320–21
Steamed Vegetables in Lemon Butter Sauce, 316–17
Stew for Two, 255
Stir-Fried Black Mushrooms with Zucchini and Chinese Greens, 327–29
Stir-Fried Lo Mein witb Shredded Vegetables, 277–78
Stomach, 132
Strawberry
  –Kiwi Salad, 265
  Shake, 300
String beans, *see* Green beans
Strudel, Savory Cabbage, 315–16
Stuffed Pita Sandwich, 282–83
Sugar, 166, 172, 223
Sugar peas, *see* Snow peas
Sulfur, 137
Summer Greens with Creamy Avocado Dressing, 338–39
Sunflower seeds, 129
Sunshine, 155, 156, 174, 178
Suntan lotion, 155
Survival into the 21st Century (Kulvinskas), 93n., 126n., 136n.
Sushi, 131, 131n.
Sweet Basil Carrots, 269
Sweeteners shopping list, 223
Sweet potatoes, 129
Sweet Spaghetti Squash, 287

Tabouli, 314
Tagamet, 90
Tamari sauce, 221

Tangelos, 204
Tangerine juices for Berry Smoothie, 308
Tangerines, 190, 204
Tangy Green Coleslaw, 264
Taste buds, 65, 186
Taub, Dr. Edward A., 17–22
Tea, 100, 161–63, 196
  decaffeinated, 162
  herbal, 163
  shopping list, 223
Teeth, 131, 164
Teriyaki Broccoli, 263–64
Testicular atrophy, 166
Thalidomide, 177
Theobromine, 165
Theory of metabolic imbalance, 55–9
Third World Congress of Alternative Medicine, 143
Thyroid problems, 143
Tilden, Dr. John H., 55–6, 58
Tomato(es), 129, 207
  Energy Salad, 238
  Properly Combined Sandwich, The, 239
  Romaine Roll-ups, 318–19
  Salsa, Fresh, 290
  Vegetable-Fruit Platter, 247
Tongue, 132
Tostada, California, 289–91
Tortilla(s)
  Avotillas, 309
  Boogie, 294
  California Tostada, 289–91
  Cuke-A-Tillas, 266
  Hot Buttered Corn, 262–63
  New York Goodwich, 251–53
  Soup, 302–3
Toxemia, *see* Metabolic imbalance
Toxemia Explained (Tilden), 55
Toxic wastes, 54, 58, 59, 62, 76, 169
  theory of detoxification, 110–18
  theory of metabolic imbalance, 55–59
  see also Elimination cycle
Trall, Dr. Russell, 42
Trop, Jack D., 51
'Truth About Milk, The,' 109
Turkey, *see* Meat
Turnips, 211

Ulcers, 98, 120, 162
Ultra-Matic juicer, 197
U.S. Department of Agriculture, 141
United States Department of Agriculture Yearbook, The, 136
U.S. Senate, Select Committee on Nutrition and Human Needs, 49
University of California, Berkeley, 165
Uric acid, 132
Uricase, 132

Vegetable(s), 61, 66, 81, 115–16, 129, 147, 168, 174
  Baked Garden, 310–11
  Bollito Misto (Steamed Vegetable Platter), 319–20
  Crusty Butter-Crumb, 274–75
  Curried, 283–85
  Farmer's Chop Suey, 307
  fresh, 229
  frozen, 229
  -fruit Platter, 247
  as high-water-content food, 61, 64, 66, 81–82
  juices, *see* Juices, vegetable
  main-course salads, 224–28
  shopping list, 208–11
  Steamed, in Lemon Butter Sauce, 316
  Stir-Fried Lo Mein with Shredded, 277–78
  Stuffed Pita Sandwich, 282–83
  Toastie, 292
  Tortilla Boogie, 294
  Tortilla Soup, 302–3
  when to eat fruit after eating, 101
  see also Salad(s); *individual types of vegetables*
Vegetable bouillon and broth, 221
Vegetable fruits, 207

Vegetarian Child, The (Gross), 126n.
Vegetarianism, 129–30, 133, 135
Vegex Co., 221
Vilabambans of Ecuador, 70, 129
Vinaigrette, Zucchini with Basil, 305–6
Vinegar, 177, 230
Vitamin B_{12}, 135
'Vitamin B_{12} Content of Some Articles of Indian Diet and Effect of Cooking on It,' 136n.
'Vitamin Megadoses Can Be Harmful,' 175n.
Vitamins, 62, 94, 98, 175–76
  supplements, 167–70, 175–76
'Vitamins of the B Complex,' 136

Waerland, Are, 52
Walker, Dr. Alan, 92, 99
Walker, Dr. Norman W, 69, 140, 143, 147n., 170, 174n., 196
Walking, 152, 154–55
Water
  distilled, 71–72
  drinking, 61, 71–72, 165
  foods with a high content of, 60–73
Watercress, 211
Watermelon for Breakfast Fruit Platter, 336
Wax beans, 211
Weekly World News, 70
Weight loss, 30–31, 32, 105, 114, 118, 186, 187, 188n.
  dairy product consumption and, 144
  diets, *see* Diets
  elimination cycle's importance, to, *see* Elimination cycle
  exercise, 151–56
  food combining and, *see* Combining foods, principle of properly
  fruit consumption and, 94, 95, 299
  permanent, 28, 30–31, 32, 41–42
Wellness-oriented physician, 18
Westbrae Natural Foods, Inc., 210, 213, 215, 219, 220, 221
Whipping cream, 218
Williams-Sonoma, 219
Wine, 167
Winick, Dr. Myron, 168, 176
Work of the Digestive Glands, The (Pavlov), 74
World Review of Nutrition and Dietetics, 128

Yale University, 94
Yam Stew, 323–24
Yogurt, 145–46, 218
  Cucumber Raita, 285
Yunqing, Wu, 70

Zucchini
  with Basil Vinaigrette, 305–6
  Harvest Soup, 261–62
  Marinated Pasta Salad, 296–98
  Mediterranean Rice Salad, 247–48
  Steamed Vegetables in Lemon Butter Sauce, 316–17
  Stir-Fried Black Mushrooms with, and Chinese Greens, 327–29
  Yam Stew, 323–24